HOME POWER WORKOUT

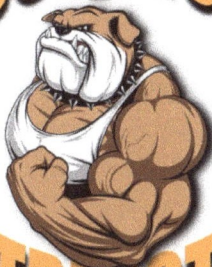

ISO QUICK STRENGTH

ISOQUICKSTRENGTH.COM

POWERLIFTING
WITH
BANDS

Table of Contents

4

About the author

Kevin's life story is a powerful testament to the resilience of the human spirit. As a writer, Kevin draws from his own experiences to share invaluable lessons on overcoming adversity and the temptation to quit. His words carry the weight of someone who has faced unimaginable challenges and emerged stronger, wiser, and more compassionate.

From a young age, Kevin's health struggles began, and he found himself facing one medical battle after another. By his 30s, he had endured a staggering 10 major medical procedures, including multiple knee operations, back surgeries, hip replacements, and treatment for an aggressive brain tumor. Even as he was writing his book, Kevin was struck by Covid-19, which led to pneumonia and daily nebulizer treatments. Lesser men might have given up, but Kevin refused to see himself as a victim of circumstance.

5

Through each diagnosis and rehabilitation, Kevin made a conscious choice to reframe adversity as an opportunity for growth. He focused on the small wins, visualizing himself healed and happy, and leaning on his deep faith and the support of loved ones during the darkest times. When fear or hopelessness crept in, he turned to prayer, uplifting books, and encouraging sayings to find the strength to take the next step forward.

As he navigated his own journey, Kevin discovered the transformative power of the mind and positive thinking. He realized that by controlling his inner world – his thoughts, beliefs, and visualizations – he could shape his outer reality. This profound insight became the foundation for his book, in which he shares his medical battles alongside the techniques he used to stay grounded in positivity.

Kevin's book is not a theoretical exploration of resilience; it is a deeply personal account of his own struggles and triumphs. He provides practical exercises to help readers overcome negative self-talk, face their fears, and visualize their desired outcomes. His message is one of hope and empowerment: no matter what life throws at us, we have the power to choose our response.

Through his writing, Kevin aims to inspire others facing their own battles to tap into their inner reserves of strength. He believes that by reframing difficulties as opportunities for growth and committing to personal development, we can overcome any obstacle, including those within our own minds.

Kevin's story is a shining example of the human capacity for resilience and the power of the human spirit. His words serve as a reminder that, no matter how many times we are knocked down, we always have the choice to get back up. In sharing his own journey, Kevin hopes to inspire others to keep going, even in the face of seemingly insurmountable odds.

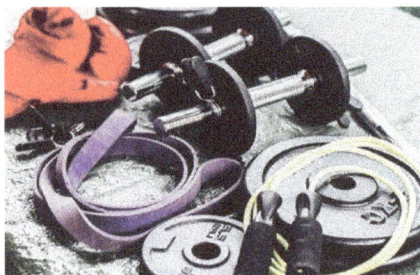

Free weight or Not to Free Weight?

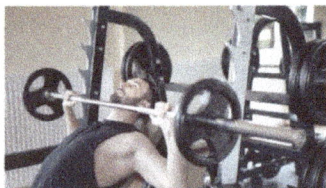

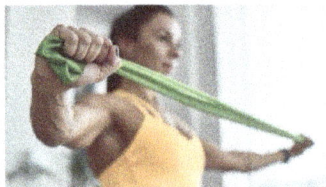

8

Chapter 1: The History and Evolution of Powerlifting: From Barbells to Resistance Bands

Powerlifting, a strength sport that has captivated athletes and fitness enthusiasts for decades, has its roots in the United States dating back to the 1950s. The sport focuses on three primary lifts: the squat, bench press, and deadlift. Competitors aim to lift the maximum weight possible in each of these exercises, with the ultimate goal of achieving the highest total combined weight across all three lifts.

The origins of powerlifting in the United States can be traced back to the 1950s, when weightlifting and bodybuilding were popular sports. However, powerlifting, which involves the competitive lifting of heavy weights in the squat, bench press, and deadlift, was not officially recognized as a sport until the 1970s.

The first organized powerlifting competition in the United States was held in 1964 in York, Pennsylvania, and was called the "York Barbell Meet." It was organized by Bob Hoffman, the founder of York Barbell Company and a key figure in the development of weightlifting and bodybuilding in the United States. This event marked a significant milestone in the history of powerlifting, as it was the first time that the three primary lifts were contested in a formal competition setting.

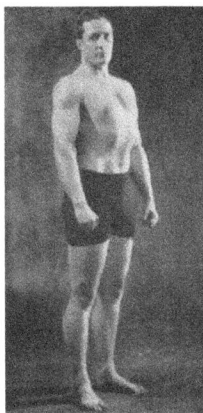

In the years following the York Barbell Meet, powerlifting began to gain traction as a distinct sport. The Amateur Athletic Union (AAU) recognized powerlifting as an official sport in 1965, and the first AAU National Powerlifting Championships were held in the same year. These events helped to establish powerlifting as a legitimate and growing sport in the United States.

As powerlifting continued to evolve, the need for a dedicated governing body became apparent. In 1972, the United States Powerlifting Federation (USPF) was formed to oversee the sport at the national level. The USPF was responsible for establishing rules and regulations, sanctioning competitions, and promoting the growth of powerlifting across the country.

On the international stage, powerlifting was also gaining recognition. The International Powerlifting Federation (IPF) was founded in 1972, bringing together powerlifting organizations from around the world. The IPF established a set of rules and regulations for international competitions, ensuring a level playing field for athletes and paving the way for the sport's continued growth and development.

Throughout the 1970s and 1980s, powerlifting continued to attract new athletes and enthusiasts. The sport's popularity was fueled by the performances of legendary lifters like Don Reinhoudt, Larry Pacifico, and Bill Kazmaier.

These athletes pushed the boundaries of human strength and set records that would stand for years to come.

One of the most iconic moments in powerlifting history occurred in 1983, when Bill Kazmaier became the first man to total over 2,400 pounds (1,089 kg) in competition. Kazmaier's incredible feat highlighted the raw power and determination of powerlifters and helped to cement the sport's place in the public consciousness.

As powerlifting entered the 1990s, the sport continued to evolve and grow. New organizations, such as the American Drug-Free Powerlifting Association (ADFPA) and the United States Powerlifting Association (USPA), were formed to promote drug-free competition and provide additional opportunities for lifters to compete.

The 1990s also saw the rise of new powerlifting superstars, such as Ed Coan and Kirk Karwoski. Ed Coan, often regarded as one of the greatest powerlifters of all time, set numerous world records across multiple weight classes throughout his career. His unparalleled strength and longevity in the sport have made him an icon and a source of inspiration for countless lifters.

Kirk Karwoski, known for his incredible squat performance, also left a lasting impact on the sport. Karwoski's intense training regimen and unrelenting drive helped him to set records and push the limits of what was thought possible in the squat. His legacy continues to inspire powerlifters to this day.

As the sport of powerlifting entered the 21st century, it continued to evolve and adapt to new challenges and opportunities. One of the most significant developments in recent years has been the increasing use of resistance bands as a training tool for powerlifters.

Resistance bands, such as pull-up bands, have become increasingly popular among powerlifters looking to add variety and specificity to their training. Unlike traditional barbells, which provide a constant level of resistance throughout the lift, resistance bands create a variable resistance that increases as the band stretches. This unique property allows lifters to target specific areas of weakness, improve explosive power, and refine their technique.

One of the primary advantages of incorporating resistance bands into powerlifting training is their versatility. Bands can be easily integrated into a wide range of exercises, from the primary lifts like squats, bench presses, and deadlifts, to accessory movements that target specific muscle groups. This versatility allows powerlifters to create highly customized training programs that address their individual needs and goals.

Accessory movements, also known as accessory exercises or assistance exercises, are supplementary exercises that target specific muscle groups to support and improve performance in the primary lifts (such as squats, bench presses, and deadlifts). These exercises

15

help address weaknesses, imbalances, and promote overall muscle development.

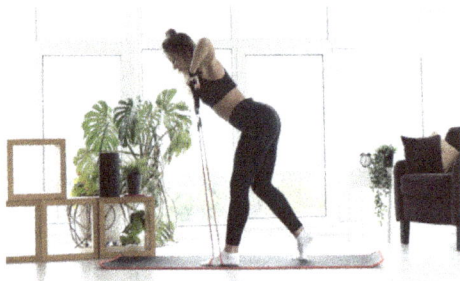

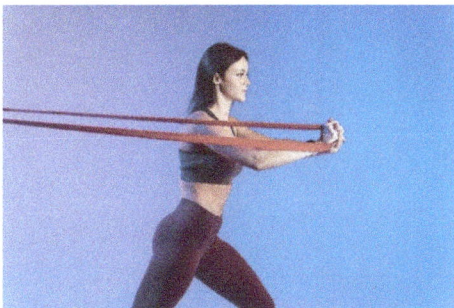

Here are some common accessory movements:

1. Pull-ups and chin-ups

2. Dips

3. Barbell rows

4. Dumbbell rows

5. Face pulls

6. Lateral raises

7. Tricep extensions

8. Bicep curls

9. Lunges

10. Glute bridges

11. Leg extensions

12. Leg curls

13. Calf raises

14. Hyperextensions

15. Planks

16. Russian twists

17. Farmer's walks

18. Suitcase carries

19. Shoulder presses

20. Push-ups

These accessory movements can be performed with various equipment, such as dumbbells, barbells, resistance bands, cables, or bodyweight. The choice of accessory exercises depends on individual goals, weaknesses, and the specific muscle groups that need additional attention to support the primary lifts and overall strength development.

Another benefit of resistance band training for powerlifters is the ability to save space and time. Unlike traditional weightlifting equipment, which can be bulky and expensive, resistance bands are compact, portable, and relatively inexpensive. This makes them an ideal option for lifters who have limited space or resources, or who need to train while traveling.

In addition to their practical benefits, resistance bands can also provide a unique training stimulus that complements traditional barbell training. By providing variable resistance throughout the lift, bands can help to increase muscle activation and improve neuromuscular control. This can lead to greater gains in strength and power over time.

When incorporating resistance bands into a powerlifting routine, it is important to start with lighter resistances and focus on proper form before progressing to heavier bands. Lifters should also be mindful of the specific strengths and weaknesses of each lift, using bands to target areas that require additional attention.

For example, in the squat, resistance bands can be used to increase the tension at the top of the movement, helping to build explosive power out of the hole. This can be particularly beneficial for lifters who struggle with the concentric phase of the lift. By attaching bands to the barbell and anchoring them to the floor, lifters can create a variable resistance that increases as they stand up from the bottom of the squat. This increased tension can help to develop the necessary speed and power to drive through the sticking point and complete the lift.

Similarly, in the bench press, bands can be used to increase the tension at the lockout, helping to build tricep strength and improve the lifter's ability to finish the lift. This can be especially useful for lifters who have difficulty with the final few inches of the press. By attaching bands to the barbell and anchoring them to the bench or power rack, lifters can create a variable resistance that increases as they press the bar to lockout. This increased tension can help to target the triceps and develop the necessary strength to complete the lift.

In the deadlift, bands can be used to increase the tension at the top of the movement, helping to build grip strength and improve lockout power. This can be particularly beneficial for lifters who struggle with maintaining their grip on heavy pulls. By attaching bands to the barbell and anchoring them to the platform, lifters can create a variable resistance that increases as they stand up with the bar. This increased tension can help to develop the necessary grip strength and lockout power to complete the lift.

Beyond the primary lifts, resistance bands can also be used to add variety and specificity to accessory movements. For example, banded face pulls can be used to target the rear deltoids and upper back, helping to improve posture and stability. To perform banded face pulls, lifters can anchor a band to a sturdy object at face level, grasp the band with both hands, and pull the band towards their face while keeping their elbows high. This movement can help to strengthen the often-neglected rear deltoids and upper back muscles, which are critical for maintaining proper posture and shoulder health. Banded face pulls are one if this authors favorite movements. A great movement for shoulders, biceps, rear deltoids, and upper back.

Banded push-ups can be used to increase the tension on the chest and triceps, providing a unique training stimulus that can lead to greater gains in size and strength. To perform banded push-ups, lifters can loop a band around their back and anchor it to a sturdy object, such as a

power rack or bench. They can then perform push-ups with the added resistance of the band, which increases as they lower their chest to the ground. This increased tension can help to target the chest and triceps muscles in a unique way, leading to greater muscle activation and growth.

Another effective use of resistance bands in powerlifting training is accommodating resistance. Accommodating resistance refers to the use of bands or chains to vary the resistance throughout the range of motion of a lift. This can be particularly useful for targeting specific areas of weakness or sticking points in a lift.

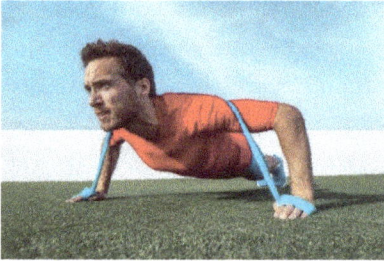

For example, in the bench press, lifters may find that they have difficulty locking out the bar at the top of the movement. By attaching bands to the barbell and anchoring them to the floor, lifters can create a variable resistance that increases as they press the bar to lockout. This increased tension at the top of the movement can help to target the triceps and develop the necessary strength to complete the lift.

Similarly, in the squat, lifters may find that they have difficulty driving out of the bottom of the movement. By attaching bands to the barbell and anchoring them to the floor, lifters can create a variable resistance that increases as they stand up from the bottom of the squat. This increased tension can help to develop speed and power.

Accommodating resistance can also be used to add variety to traditional powerlifting exercises. For example, banded deadlifts can be performed by attaching a band to the barbell and anchoring it to the platform. As the lifter stands up with the bar, the band tension increases, providing a unique challenge to the posterior chain muscles. This variation can be particularly useful for lifters who have reached a plateau in their traditional deadlift training. Note: I have developed the lying deadlift. To save my hips and back, I lay on the floor with the band anchored to a pole or wall at around the top of my foot. Stretch the band to a good tension, then bend at the torso. The exact same movement as a standing deadlift with much less tension on hips, knees and back.

Another effective use of resistance bands in powerlifting training is for warm-up and activation exercises. Bands can be used to perform a variety of dynamic stretches and movement drills that can help to prepare the body for heavy lifting.

For example, banded leg swings can be used to dynamically stretch the hip flexors and hamstrings, while also activating the glutes and core muscles. To perform banded leg swings, lifters can loop a band around a sturdy object and place one foot inside the band. They can then swing their leg forward and back, focusing on maintaining a stable core and keeping their knee slightly bent.

Similarly, banded pull-aparts can be used to activate the upper back and shoulder muscles prior to bench pressing or overhead pressing. To perform banded pull-aparts, lifters can grasp a band with both hands and pull the band apart while keeping their arms straight. This movement can help to engage the rear deltoids, rhomboids, and other upper back muscles, which are critical for maintaining proper shoulder positioning during pressing exercises.

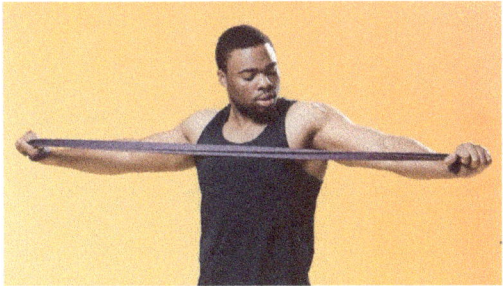

Resistance bands can also be used for injury prevention and rehabilitation purposes in powerlifting. By providing a low-impact, variable resistance training stimulus, bands can help lifters to safely strengthen and stabilize injured or weakened areas of the body.

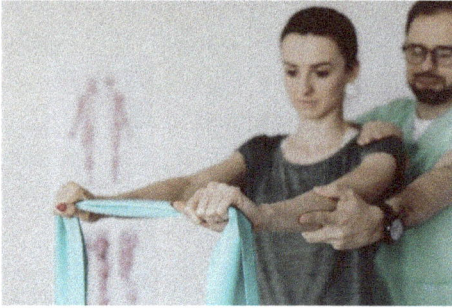

For example, lifters who have experienced knee pain or injury may benefit from incorporating banded squats or leg extensions into their training. By providing resistance without the compressive forces of traditional barbell squats, these exercises can help to safely strengthen the quadriceps and other knee-supporting muscles.

Similarly, lifters who have experienced shoulder pain or injury may benefit from incorporating banded external rotations or face pulls into their training. These exercises can help to strengthen the rotator cuff and other shoulder-stabilizing muscles, which are critical for maintaining proper shoulder health and function.

In addition to their use in specific exercises, resistance bands can also be used to create full-body training circuits that challenge the cardiovascular system and burn fat. By combining exercises like banded squats, push-ups, rows, and jumps, lifters can create high-intensity, full-body workouts that provide a unique challenge to the muscles and cardiovascular system.

For example, a sample resistance band circuit workout might include the following exercises:

1. Banded Squats x 20 reps

2. Banded Push-Ups x 15 reps

3. Banded Rows x 15 reps

4. Banded Jumps x 30 seconds

Lifters can perform each exercise for the prescribed number of reps or time, then move immediately to the next exercise with minimal rest between sets. This type of high-intensity, full-body training can be particularly useful for lifters who are looking to improve their overall conditioning and burn extra fat.

Another benefit of resistance band training for powerlifters is the ability to perform exercises in multiple planes of motion. Traditional barbell exercises like squats, bench presses, and deadlifts are primarily performed in the sagittal plane (front-to-back). However, resistance bands can be used to perform exercises in the frontal plane (side-to-side) and transverse plane (rotational), which can help to improve overall athleticism and reduce the risk of injury.

For example, banded lateral walks can be used to target the hip abductors and glutes in the frontal plane. To perform banded lateral walks, lifters can place a band around their ankles or just above their knees, then step laterally while maintaining tension on the band. This exercise can help to improve hip stability and reduce the risk of knee injuries.

Similarly, banded rotational chops can be used to target the core muscles in the transverse plane. To perform banded rotational chops, lifters can anchor a band to a sturdy object at shoulder height, then grasp the band with both hands and rotate their torso while keeping their arms straight. This exercise can help to improve rotational power and stability, which can translate to improved performance in the squat and deadlift.

Finally, resistance bands can be used to create custom training tools and accessories that can help powerlifters to target specific areas of weakness or perform exercises with greater specificity.

For example, lifters can create their own banded hamstring curl by looping a band around their feet and anchoring it to a sturdy object. They can then lie face down and curl their heels towards their glutes against the resistance of the band. This exercise can be particularly useful for lifters who have difficulty targeting their hamstrings with traditional exercises like lying leg curls.

Similarly, lifters can create their own banded hip thrust by looping a band around their hips and anchoring it to a sturdy object behind them. They can then lie face up with their upper back supported on a bench and thrust their hips towards the ceiling against the resistance of the band. This exercise can be particularly useful for lifters who want to target their glutes with greater specificity than traditional barbell hip thrusts.

In conclusion, resistance bands offer a wide range of benefits for powerlifters looking to improve their strength, power, and overall performance. From their versatility and cost-effectiveness to their ability to target specific areas of weakness and provide accommodating resistance, bands are a valuable tool that every powerlifter should consider incorporating into their training.

As the sport of powerlifting continues to evolve and grow, it is likely that we will see even more innovative uses of resistance bands and other alternative training methods. By staying open-minded and experimenting with new techniques and tools, powerlifters can continue to push the boundaries of what is possible and take their strength and performance to new heights.

Ultimately, the key to success in powerlifting is not just about lifting heavy weights, but about finding the training methods and tools that work best for your individual needs and goals. Whether you are a seasoned competitor or a beginner just starting out, resistance bands can help you to unlock your full potential and achieve your powerlifting dreams. So why not try them and see how they can take your training to the next level?

Chapter 2: Introduction to Powerlifting with Resistance Bands

Benefits of Powerlifting with Resistance Bands

Powerlifting with resistance bands offers a dynamic and versatile approach to enhancing strength and targeting individual muscle groups with precision. By providing consistent resistance throughout each movement, bands engage and fortify muscles, leading to greater gains in strength and overall athletic performance. The unique properties of resistance bands allow for a more targeted and efficient workout, as the resistance increases as the bands stretch, challenging muscles at their strongest points.

In addition to their effectiveness, resistance bands are portable and versatile, making them ideal for individuals who may not have access to a gym or prefer to work out at home. They offer a cost-effective and space-saving alternative to traditional weightlifting equipment, allowing for a comprehensive workout routine that can be easily adapted to suit individual needs and goals.

Moreover, incorporating resistance bands into your powerlifting routine enhances stability, balance, and coordination while strengthening smaller, often neglected muscle groups. This comprehensive approach to training not only boosts performance in powerlifting and other sports but also plays a crucial role in preventing injuries and promoting overall physical well-being. By targeting stabilizer muscles and improving joint stability, resistance bands help to create a more balanced and resilient body, reducing the risk of common injuries associated with powerlifting.

The versatility of resistance bands also allows for a wide range of exercises and variations, enabling lifters to target specific muscle groups and address individual weaknesses. By incorporating different band tensions, attachment points, and body positions, lifters can create an endless array of challenges to keep their workouts engaging and effective. This variety helps to prevent plateaus and keeps the body adapting to new stimuli, leading to continuous progress and gains.

Furthermore, resistance bands provide accommodating resistance, meaning that the resistance increases as the bands stretch, making the exercise more challenging at the end of the range of motion where the muscle is strongest. This unique feature of resistance bands helps to develop power and explosiveness, which are critical components of successful powerlifting performance. By training with accommodating resistance, lifters can improve their ability to generate force quickly and efficiently, translating to improved performance on the platform.

In addition to the physical benefits, powerlifting with resistance bands also offers mental and psychological advantages. The convenience and accessibility of resistance bands make it easier to maintain a consistent workout routine, promoting discipline and adherence to training. The ability to work out anytime, anywhere, eliminates many of the barriers and excuses that can derail progress. Moreover, the visible progress and increased strength that come from consistent training with resistance bands can boost confidence and self-esteem, enhancing overall well-being and mental resilience.

Overall, powerlifting with resistance bands is a valuable tool for individuals looking to build strength, power, and muscle mass. Whether you

37

are a beginner or an experienced lifter, incorporating resistance bands into your routine can help you achieve your fitness goals and take your training to new heights. With consistent use, resistance bands can improve muscular endurance, enhance stability, and balance, and target specific muscle groups with greater precision. By embracing the unique challenges and benefits of resistance band training, lifters can unlock their full potential and maximize their performance both in the gym and on the platform.

Overview of Powerlifting Techniques

Powerlifting is a strength sport that focuses on three main lifts: the squat, bench press, and deadlift. These lifts require a combination of strength, technique, and mental focus to execute properly. In this subchapter, we will provide an in-depth overview of powerlifting techniques, specifically focusing on how resistance bands can be used to enhance your training and optimize your performance.

Form and technique are paramount in powerlifting, as they not only ensure the safety of the lifter but also maximize the effectiveness of each lift. Maintaining a neutral spine, engaging the core, and utilizing proper breathing techniques are fundamental principles that apply to all powerlifting movements. Resistance bands can be incredibly useful in reinforcing these techniques and providing instant feedback on form.

When incorporated into powerlifting exercises, resistance bands offer a unique form of feedback that can help lifters identify and correct technical inefficiencies. For example, when squatting with a band around the knees, lifters can feel the band's tension increase if their knees cave inward, providing an immediate cue to correct the issue. Similarly, using bands during bench press can help lifters maintain proper elbow position and prevent excessive flaring, reducing the risk of shoulder injuries.

In addition to providing feedback on form, resistance bands can also be used to address specific weaknesses and imbalances in powerlifting techniques. By strategically placing bands to target certain phases of the lift, lifters can overload specific muscle groups and movement patterns, leading to improved strength and technical proficiency. For instance, using bands to increase resistance at the bottom of the squat can help lifters develop explosive power out of the hole, while banded deadlifts can improve lockout strength and hip extension.

Understanding the biomechanics of each lift is another crucial aspect of powerlifting technique, and resistance bands can be a valuable tool in developing this understanding. By providing variable resistance throughout the range of motion, bands can help lifters identify and strengthen weak points in their technique. This is particularly useful for lifters who struggle with certain phases of the lift, such as the sticking point in the bench press or the initial pull off the floor in the deadlift.

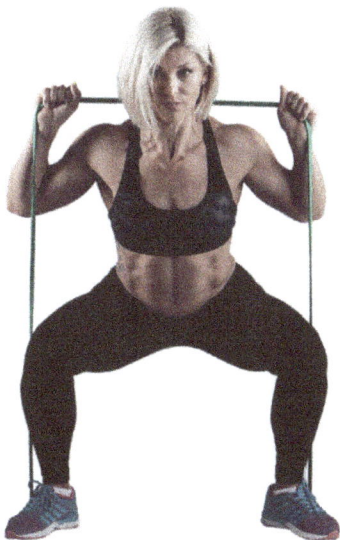

Moreover, resistance bands can be used to increase the intensity and specificity of powerlifting training. By adding bands to traditional barbell exercises, lifters can create a more challenging and sport-specific stimulus, as the accommodating resistance provided by the bands more closely mimics the demands of powerlifting competition. This can help lifters develop the specific strength and power needed to excel on the platform.

Resistance bands also offer a way to safely overload powerlifting movements and push past plateaus. By using bands to increase resistance at the top of the lift, where the lifter is strongest, lifters can safely handle heavier loads and develop maximal strength without the risk of injury associated with excessively heavy barbell training. This can be particularly beneficial for lifters who have reached a plateau in their traditional powerlifting training and need a novel stimulus to continue making progress.

Beyond their applications in the three main powerlifting movements, resistance bands can also be used to improve overall athleticism and support long-term powerlifting success. Incorporating banded exercises that target the posterior chain, such as banded good mornings and hip thrusts, can help to build the strength and stability needed to maintain proper form under heavy loads. Additionally, using bands for accessory exercises like pull-ups, rows, and face pulls can help to balance out the pushing movements that dominate powerlifting training, promoting shoulder health, and reducing the risk of injury.

Overall, powerlifting techniques can be greatly enhanced through the strategic use of resistance bands. By providing feedback on form, addressing specific weaknesses, increasing training intensity, and promoting overall athleticism, bands can help lifters of all levels take their powerlifting performance to new heights. Whether used as a primary training tool or as a complement to traditional barbell training, resistance bands are a valuable asset in the pursuit of powerlifting mastery.

How Resistance Bands Can Enhance Powerlifting Performance

Resistance bands have become increasingly popular among powerlifters looking to enhance their performance and take their training to the next level. These versatile tools offer a unique form of resistance that can complement traditional barbell training and provide a range of benefits for strength, power, and technical development. By understanding the specific ways in which resistance bands can enhance powerlifting performance, lifters can effectively integrate them into their training programs and maximize their gains.

One of the primary benefits of resistance bands is their ability to provide accommodating resistance. Unlike traditional free weights, which provide a constant level of resistance throughout the lift, resistance bands increase in tension as they stretch. This means that the resistance is greatest at the end range of motion, where the muscle is in its strongest position. By challenging the muscle at its peak contraction, resistance bands can help to develop explosive power and improve the ability to generate force quickly, which is critical for success in powerlifting.

Accommodating resistance is particularly beneficial for developing sticking point strength in the powerlifting movements. Many lifters struggle with specific portions of the lift, such as the transition from the chest to the lockout in the bench press or the mid-range of the deadlift. By using resistance bands to overload these specific areas, lifters can target their weaknesses and build the strength needed to power through sticking points. This can lead to significant improvements in performance and the ability to handle heavier loads.

In addition to providing accommodating resistance, resistance bands can also be used to increase the overall intensity of powerlifting training. By adding bands to traditional barbell exercises, lifters can create a more challenging stimulus that forces the muscles to work harder and adapt to new demands. This increased intensity can help to break through plateaus and spark new gains in strength and muscle mass.

Another way in which resistance bands can enhance powerlifting performance is by promoting proper form. When used correctly, resistance bands provide instant feedback on movement quality and can help lifters identify and correct technical inefficiencies. For example, when squatting with a band around the knees, lifters can feel the band's tension increase if their knees cave inward, cueing them to drive their knees outward and maintain proper alignment. Similarly, using bands during bench press can help lifters maintain proper elbow position and prevent excessive flaring, reducing the risk of shoulder injuries.

Resistance bands can also be used to develop specific qualities that are critical for powerlifting success, such as stability, control, and body awareness. By incorporating banded exercises that challenge balance and proprioception, such as banded single-leg squats or banded push-ups, lifters can improve their overall body control and develop the stability needed to maintain proper form under heavy loads. This can translate to improved performance on the platform and a reduced risk of injury.

In addition to their direct applications in the powerlifting movements, resistance bands can also be used to enhance overall athleticism and support long-term powerlifting success. Incorporating banded exercises that target the posterior chain, such as banded good mornings and hip thrusts, can help to build the strength and stability needed to maintain proper form under heavy loads. Additionally, using bands for accessory exercises like pull-ups, rows, and face pulls can help to balance out the pushing movements that dominate powerlifting training, promoting shoulder health, and reducing the risk of injury.

Furthermore, resistance bands offer a low-impact alternative to traditional barbell training, which can be beneficial for powerlifters looking to manage stress and prevent overuse injuries. By incorporating banded exercises into their training programs, lifters can maintain strength and muscle mass while reducing the overall stress on their joints and connective tissues. This can be particularly useful during deload periods or when recovering from injuries.

Finally, resistance bands provide a versatile and convenient training option for powerlifters who may have limited access to equipment or who prefer to train at home. With a simple set of bands, lifters can perform a wide range of exercises that target all of the major muscle groups and support their powerlifting goals. This flexibility can be invaluable for lifters who travel frequently or who have busy schedules that make it difficult to consistently access a fully equipped gym.

In conclusion, resistance bands are a powerful tool for enhancing powerlifting performance and supporting long-term success in the sport. By providing accommodating resistance, increasing training intensity, promoting proper form, developing specific qualities, enhancing overall athleticism, offering a low-impact alternative to barbell training, and providing a convenient training option, resistance bands can help powerlifters of all levels take their training and performance to new heights.

To maximize the benefits of resistance band training, powerlifters should work with a qualified coach or trainer to develop a comprehensive program that integrates bands into their existing routine. This may involve using bands as a primary training tool for certain exercises or incorporating them as a complement to traditional barbell training. Regardless of the specific approach, the key is to use bands strategically and progressively, gradually increasing the resistance and complexity of the exercises over time.

In addition to using bands in their own training, powerlifters can also benefit from incorporating them into their warm-up and recovery routines. Using bands for dynamic stretching and activation exercises can help to improve mobility, increase blood flow, and prepare the body for the demands of heavy lifting. Similarly, using bands for post-workout recovery exercises like banded leg curls or banded pull-aparts can help to promote relaxation and reduce muscle soreness.

Ultimately, the key to success with resistance band training is consistency and patience. Like any form of training, the benefits of resistance bands will accumulate over time with regular practice and progressive overload. By staying committed to their training and continually challenging themselves with new variations and resistances, powerlifters can use resistance bands to unlock their full potential and achieve their goals in the sport.

In summary, resistance bands are a valuable tool for powerlifters looking to enhance their performance and take their training to the next level. By providing accommodating resistance, increasing training intensity, promoting proper form, developing specific qualities, enhancing overall athleticism, offering a low-impact alternative to barbell training, and providing a convenient training option, resistance bands can help powerlifters of all levels achieve their goals and succeed on the platform. Whether used as a primary training tool or as a complement to traditional barbell training, resistance bands are an essential piece of equipment for any serious powerlifter.

How resistance bands can mimic powerlifting movements

Resistance bands have become increasingly popular in the world of strength training, and for good reason. These versatile tools can be used to mimic a wide range of exercises, including the three main powerlifting movements: the squat, bench press, and deadlift. By understanding how resistance bands can be used to replicate these movements, lifters can incorporate them into their training programs and reap the numerous benefits they offer.

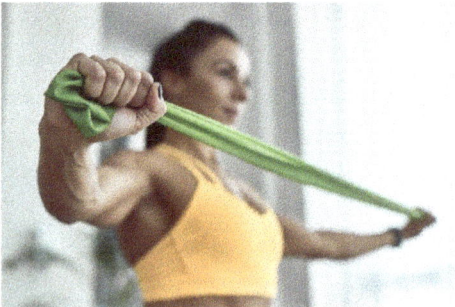

One of the most significant advantages of using resistance bands to mimic powerlifting movements is their ability to provide accommodating resistance. Unlike traditional free weights, which provide a constant level of resistance throughout the lift, resistance bands increase in tension as they stretch. This means that the resistance is greatest at the end range of motion, where the muscle is in its strongest position. By challenging the muscle at its peak contraction, resistance bands can help to develop explosive power and improve the ability to generate force quickly, which is critical for success in powerlifting.

When using resistance bands to mimic the squat, lifters can attach a band to a secure anchor point and loop it around their shoulders, creating a similar resistance profile to a barbell squat. As the lifter descends into the squat, the band tension increases, providing a greater challenge to the quadriceps, glutes, and hamstrings. This increased tension at the bottom of the squat can help to develop strength and power out of the hole, which is often a sticking point for many lifters.

Similarly, resistance bands can be used to mimic the bench press by attaching them to a secure anchor point and looping them around the lifter's hands or wrists. As the lifter presses the bands away from their chest, the tension increases, providing a similar resistance profile to a barbell bench press. This increased tension at the top of the lift can help to develop lockout strength and improve the ability to generate force quickly, which is critical for success in powerlifting.

For the deadlift, resistance bands can be attached to a secure anchor point and looped around the lifter's feet or ankles. As the lifter pulls the bands up and away from the ground, the tension increases, providing a similar resistance profile to a barbell deadlift. This increased tension at the top of the lift can help to develop lockout strength and improve the ability to generate force quickly, which is critical for success in powerlifting.

In addition to providing accommodating resistance, resistance bands can also be used to increase the overall intensity of powerlifting training. By adding bands to traditional barbell exercises, lifters can create a more challenging stimulus that forces the muscles to work harder and adapt to new demands. This increased intensity can help to break through plateaus and spark new gains in strength and muscle mass.

Another benefit of using resistance bands to mimic powerlifting movements is their ability to promote ideal body placement and control. When used correctly, resistance bands provide instant feedback on movement quality and can help lifters identify and correct technical inefficiencies. For example, when squatting with a band around the knees, lifters can feel the band's tension increase if their knees cave inward, cueing them to drive their knees outward and maintain proper alignment. Similarly, using bands during bench press can help lifters maintain proper elbow position and prevent excessive flaring, reducing the risk of shoulder injuries.

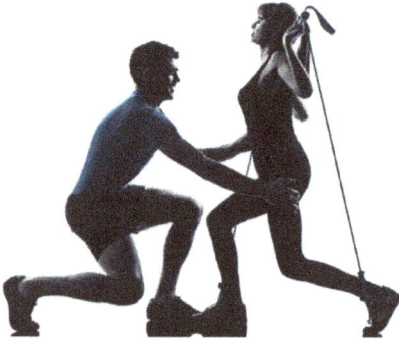

Resistance bands can also be used to develop specific qualities that are critical for powerlifting success, such as stability, control, and body awareness. By incorporating banded exercises that challenge balance and proprioception, such as banded single-leg squats or banded push-ups, lifters can improve their overall body control and develop the stability needed to maintain proper form under heavy loads. This can translate to improved performance on the platform and a reduced risk of injury.

Furthermore, resistance bands offer a low-impact alternative to traditional barbell training, which can be beneficial for powerlifters looking to manage stress and prevent overuse injuries. By incorporating banded exercises into their training programs, lifters can maintain strength and muscle mass while reducing the overall stress on their joints and connective tissues. This can be particularly useful during deload periods or when recovering from injuries.

Finally, resistance bands provide a versatile and convenient training option for powerlifters who may have limited access to equipment or who prefer to train at home. With a simple set of bands, lifters can perform a wide range of exercises that target all the major muscle groups and support their powerlifting goals. This flexibility can be invaluable for lifters who travel frequently or who have busy schedules that make it difficult to consistently access a fully equipped gym.

To effectively incorporate resistance bands into powerlifting training, lifters should start by mastering the basic movement patterns with bodyweight or light resistance. Once form and technique have been established, lifters can gradually increase the resistance by using thicker bands or adding additional bands to the setup. It is important to progress slowly and listen to the body, as adding too much resistance too quickly can lead to injury or technical breakdown.

When using resistance bands to mimic powerlifting movements, lifters should also pay close attention to their setup and execution. Proper band placement and anchoring are critical for ensuring safety and effectiveness, as a poorly secured band can snap or slip during the lift, leading to injury. Lifters should also focus on maintaining precise alignment and motion throughout the entire range of motion.

Chapter 3: Understanding Resistance Bands

Types of Resistance Bands (HEAVY DUTY PULL UP BANDS)

When it comes to powerlifting with resistance bands, selecting the right type of band is paramount to achieving your desired results. Heavy-duty pull-up bands are a popular choice among powerlifters due to their ability to provide maximum resistance, making them ideal for building strength and power.

These high-quality latex rubber bands come in various resistance levels, ranging from light to extra heavy. The resistance level is determined by the band's thickness and width, with thicker and wider bands offering more resistance. This allows powerlifters to choose the appropriate level of resistance based on their current strength and fitness goals.

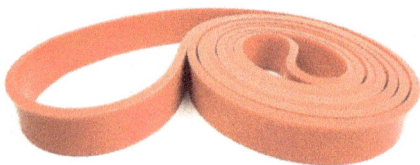

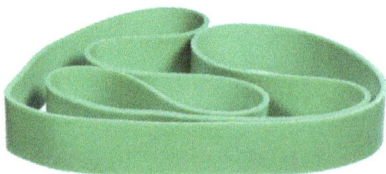

One of the key advantages of heavy-duty pull-up bands is their versatility. They can be incorporated into a wide array of exercises, such as pull-ups, squats, deadlifts, and bench presses. By using these bands, powerlifters can increase the intensity of their workouts and challenge their muscles in new and innovative ways. This targeted approach helps to develop specific muscle groups with precision, leading to improved overall strength and power.

When selecting a heavy-duty pull-up band, it is essential to consider your current strength level and fitness objectives. Beginners may want to start with a lighter resistance band and gradually progress to heavier bands as they build strength and confidence. It is also crucial to properly maintain and store your bands to ensure their longevity and effectiveness. This includes keeping them away from extreme temperatures, cleaning them regularly, and inspecting them for signs of wear and tear.

Incorporating heavy-duty pull-up bands into your powerlifting routine can be a meaningful change. These bands allow you to increase resistance, target specific muscle groups, and achieve greater strength and power gains. By selecting the appropriate band for your needs and properly caring for it, you can take your powerlifting performance to new heights.

Choosing the Right Resistance Bands for Powerlifting

Selecting the appropriate resistance bands is a critical factor in maximizing your strength and power gains in powerlifting. With a wide variety of options available on the market, it can be overwhelming to determine which bands best suit your needs. To help you make an informed decision, consider the following factors.

1. Resistance level: Resistance bands come in various levels of resistance, ranging from light to

heavy. It is essential to select bands that provide sufficient resistance to challenge your muscles without causing strain or injury. If you are new to powerlifting or resistance band training, it is recommended to start with lighter bands and gradually increase the resistance as you build strength and confidence. This approach allows your body to adapt to the new stimulus and reduces the risk of injury.

2. Length and width: When it comes to powerlifting exercises, opt for longer and wider bands. These bands offer more stability and support during heavy lifts, ensuring that you can maintain form and technique throughout the movement. Additionally, choose bands made of durable, high-quality materials that can withstand the rigors of powerlifting workouts. This will help to extend the life of your bands and provide consistent resistance over time.

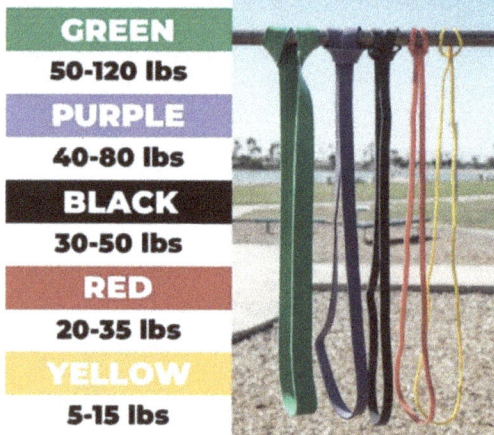

GREEN	50-120 lbs
PURPLE	40-80 lbs
BLACK	30-50 lbs
RED	20-35 lbs
YELLOW	5-15 lbs

3. Versatility: While some resistance bands are designed for specific exercises, others can be used for a variety of movements. When selecting bands for powerlifting, look for options that can be easily incorporated into your existing routine and provide resistance for different muscle groups. This versatility allows you to target multiple areas of your body and keeps your workouts engaging and effective.

4. Budget: Resistance bands are available at various price points, so it is important to find bands that fit within your budget while still meeting your strength and power gain requirements. Keep in mind that investing in high-quality bands may cost more upfront but can save you money in the long run by lasting longer and providing more consistent resistance.

Before starting any new exercise program, it is always recommended to consult with a professional trainer or coach. They can help you select the appropriate resistance bands for your needs, demonstrate proper form and technique, and create a personalized training plan that aligns with your goals and fitness level. By working with a qualified professional, you can ensure that you are using resistance bands safely and effectively to maximize your powerlifting performance.

Proper Care and Maintenance of Bands

Investing in resistance bands is an excellent way to enhance your powerlifting routine, but to ensure that your bands remain in top condition and continue to provide effective workouts, proper care and maintenance are essential. By following these simple tips, you can extend the life of your resistance bands and get the most out of your investment:

1. Storage: After each use, it is crucial to store your resistance bands properly. Avoid leaving them exposed to direct sunlight or extreme temperatures, as this can cause the material to degrade and lose its elasticity over time. Instead, store your bands in a cool, dry place, such as a drawer or a dedicated storage bag. This will help to prevent damage and ensure that your bands are ready to use whenever you need them.

2. Cleaning: Resistance bands can accumulate sweat, dirt, and bacteria over time, which can lead to unpleasant odors and potential health

risks. To keep your bands clean and hygienic, make sure to wipe them down with a damp cloth or a mild cleaning solution after each use. This simple step will remove any buildup and keep your bands fresh for your next workout. Avoid using harsh chemicals or abrasive materials, as these can damage the band's surface and compromise its integrity.

3. Inspection: Before each use, take a moment to inspect your resistance bands for signs of wear and tear. Look for any fraying, cracking, or stretching, which may indicate that the band is weakening and could potentially snap during use. If you notice any damage, it is best to err on the side of caution and replace the band to prevent injury. Regular inspections can help you identify potential issues early on and ensure that you are always working with safe and reliable equipment.

4. Proper use: To maximize the lifespan of your resistance bands and prevent unnecessary damage, it is essential to use them correctly. Always follow the manufacturer's instructions and

guidelines for safe use and avoid stretching the bands beyond their intended capacity. When anchoring your bands, make sure to use sturdy, secure attachment points that can withstand the tension and pressure of your workouts. Avoid exposing your bands to sharp edges or abrasive surfaces, as this can cause cuts or tears in the material.

5. Replacement: Despite your best efforts to care for and maintain your resistance bands, they will eventually wear out and lose their effectiveness over time. The lifespan of a resistance band can vary depending on factors such as the quality of the material, frequency of use, and storage conditions. As a rule of thumb, it is recommended to replace your bands every 6 to 12 months, or sooner if you notice any significant signs of wear and tear. By replacing your bands regularly, you can ensure that you are always working with safe, reliable equipment that provides optimal resistance and support for your powerlifting goals.

In addition to these care and maintenance tips, it is also important to educate yourself on the proper use and safety guidelines for resistance bands. Always start with a lighter resistance and gradually increase the intensity as you build strength and confidence. Make sure to maintain great form throughout each exercise and stop immediately if you experience any pain or discomfort. If you are unsure about how to use your resistance bands correctly, seek guidance from a qualified fitness professional or consult reliable resources such as instructional videos or guides.

By taking the time to properly care for and maintain your resistance bands, you can ensure that they remain a valuable and effective tool in your powerlifting arsenal. Not only will this help to extend the life of your bands and save you money in the long run, but it will also allow you to continue challenging yourself and making progress toward your strength and power goals. Remember, investing in your equipment is an

investment in yourself and your powerlifting
journey.

Chapter 4: Essential Powerlifting Techniques

Squatting with Resistance Bands

Squatting with resistance bands is a highly effective technique for powerlifters looking to take their training to the next level. By incorporating resistance bands into your squat routine, you can target your leg muscles in ways that traditional barbell squats cannot, leading to increased strength, improved stability, and enhanced overall performance.

The primary muscles targeted during squats with resistance bands are the quadriceps,

hamstrings, and glutes. The quadriceps, located on the front of your thighs, are responsible for extending your knees and are heavily engaged during the concentric (upward) phase of the squat. The hamstrings, found on the back of your

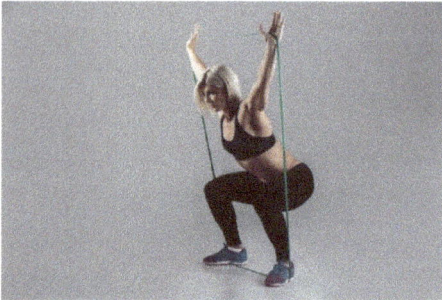

thighs, work in conjunction with your glutes to extend your hips and provide stability throughout the movement. Your glutes, the largest muscle group in your body, play a crucial role in hip extension and are heavily recruited during the squat.

To perform squats with resistance bands, start by securing the bands under your feet and holding the handles at shoulder height. Stand with your feet shoulder-width apart, engage your core, and keep your chest up. As you descend into the squat, focus on maintaining tension in the bands by pushing your knees outward. This will help activate your glutes and ensure proper form throughout the movement.

As you reach the bottom of the squat, pause for a moment, and feel the tension in your legs. The resistance bands should provide constant tension, challenging your muscles throughout the entire range of motion. From this position, drive through your heels and extend your hips and knees to return to the starting position.

One of the key benefits of squatting with resistance bands is the increased time under tension. Unlike traditional barbell squats, where the resistance is only present during the concentric phase, resistance bands provide constant tension throughout the entire movement. This increased time under tension leads to greater muscle activation and can help stimulate muscle growth and strength development.

Another advantage of using resistance bands for squats is the added stability challenge. As you move through the squat, the bands will try to pull you forward or backward, forcing your stabilizing muscles to work overtime to maintain proper form. This increased stability challenge can help improve your balance, coordination, and overall body control, translating to better performance in other powerlifting movements.

In addition to the primary leg muscles targeted during squats, using resistance bands also engages your core and upper body. Your core muscles, including your abdominal muscles, obliques, and lower back, work to stabilize your spine and maintain proper posture throughout the movement. Your upper back and shoulder muscles are also engaged as you hold the handles at shoulder height, providing additional stability and support.

To maximize the benefits of squatting with resistance bands, it is important to focus on proper form and technique. Start with a lighter resistance band and focus on maintaining tension throughout the entire movement. As you become more comfortable with the exercise, gradually increase the resistance to continue challenging your muscles.

Incorporating squats with resistance bands into your powerlifting routine can be a game-changer for your leg strength and overall performance. Whether you are using them as a primary squat variation or as an accessory movement to complement your barbell squats, the added resistance and stability challenge provided by the bands can help take your training to the next level.

Banded Squats

Banded squats are a powerful exercise that can help powerlifters build explosive strength, improve stability, and enhance overall performance. By adding resistance bands to your squat routine, you can challenge your muscles in new ways and take your training to the next level.

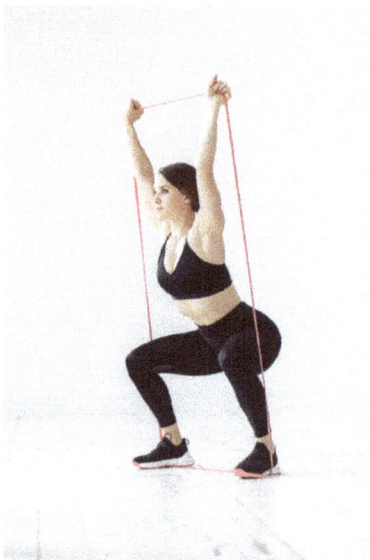

The primary muscles targeted during banded squats are the same as traditional squats – the quadriceps, hamstrings, and glutes. However, the addition of resistance bands provides a unique challenge that can help further engage these muscle groups and lead to greater strength gains.

To perform banded squats, start by securing a resistance band to a sturdy anchor point, such as a power rack or squat stand. Step inside the band and position it just above your knees. Set up for your squat as you normally would, with your feet shoulder-width apart and your chest up.

As you descend into the squat, the resistance band will provide accommodating resistance, meaning the tension will increase as you move deeper into the squat. This increased tension forces your muscles to work harder, particularly in the bottom portion of the movement where many lifters struggle.

The accommodating resistance provided by the bands also helps to improve your explosiveness out of the hole. As you drive up from the bottom of the squat, the bands will provide additional resistance, forcing your muscles to contract more forcefully to overcome the added tension. This can translate to improved power and speed in your traditional barbell squats.

In addition to providing accommodating resistance, banded squats also challenge your stability and balance. As you move through the squat, the bands will try to pull you forward or backward, engaging your stabilizing muscles to keep you upright and in proper form. This increased stability challenge can help improve your overall body control and reduce your risk of injury.

Banded squats also provide a unique stimulus for your hip extensors, particularly your glutes. As you drive out of the bottom of the squat, the bands will try to pull your knees inward, forcing your glutes to work harder to keep your knees in line with your toes. This increased glute activation can help build strength and power in your posterior chain, which is crucial for powerlifting performance.

When performing banded squats, it is important to maintain perfect form. Keep your chest up, your core engaged, and your weight evenly distributed throughout your feet. Focus on driving your knees outward to maintain tension on the bands and avoid letting them pull you forward or backward.

As with any new exercise, start with a lighter resistance band and focus on perfecting your form before adding more tension. As you become more comfortable with the movement, gradually increase the resistance to continue challenging your muscles and driving progress.

Incorporating banded squats into your powerlifting routine can be a powerful tool for building strength, improving stability, and enhancing overall performance. Whether you use them as a primary squat variation or as an accessory movement to complement your traditional barbell squats, the unique challenges provided by the bands can help take your training to the next level.

Variations (e.g., front squats, pause squats)

While traditional back squats are a staple in most powerlifting routines, incorporating variations like front squats and pause squats can help target specific muscle groups, improve weaknesses, and add variety to your training.

Front squats are a variation that places greater emphasis on the quadriceps and upper back compared to traditional back squats. To perform front squats with resistance bands, set up the bands as you would for banded back squats, but instead of positioning the bar on your upper back, hold it across your shoulders with your elbows pointing forward.

The front rack position required for front squats places a greater demand on your upper back and core muscles to maintain proper posture throughout the movement. This can help improve your overall stability and reduce your risk of injury in other powerlifting movements.

Front squats also target your quadriceps more directly than back squats, making them an excellent accessory movement for lifters looking to improve their leg strength and hypertrophy. The added resistance from the bands can help increase the difficulty of the movement, leading to greater muscle activation and growth.

Pause squats are another variation that can be enhanced with the use of resistance bands. To perform banded pause squats, set up as you would for traditional banded squats, but add a pause at the bottom of the movement before driving back up to the starting position.

The pause at the bottom of the squat eliminates the stretch reflex and forces your muscles to

81

generate force from a dead stop. This can help improve your strength and power out of the hole, which is often a sticking point for many lifters.

Pause squats also place a greater demand on your core and stabilizing muscles, as you must maintain tension throughout the pause to avoid collapsing or losing form. This increased stability challenge can translate to improved control and technique in your other powerlifting movements.

When performing banded pause squats, focus on maintaining tension in your muscles throughout the pause. Avoid relaxing or letting your form break down, as this can reduce the effectiveness of the exercise and increase your risk of injury.

As with any squat variation, start with a lighter resistance band and focus on maintaining proper form before adding more tension. Gradually increase the duration of your pause as you become more comfortable with the movement, working up to a 2-3 second pause in the bottom position.

Incorporating front squats and pause squats with resistance bands into your powerlifting routine can help target specific muscle groups, address weaknesses, and improve overall performance. By adding variety to your training and challenging your muscles in new ways, you can continue to make progress and reach your strength and hypertrophy goals.

Banded Bench Press

The bench press is one of the three primary lifts in powerlifting, targeting the chest, shoulders, and triceps. Incorporating resistance bands into your bench press routine can help increase the difficulty of the movement, leading to greater strength gains and improved performance.

The primary muscles targeted during the bench press are the pectoralis major (chest), anterior deltoids (front shoulders), and triceps brachii (back of the upper arm). The pectoralis major is the large, fan-shaped muscle that makes up the bulk of the chest and is primarily responsible for horizontal adduction of the arm (bringing the arm across the body). The anterior deltoids are located on the front of the shoulder and assist in shoulder flexion and horizontal adduction. The triceps brachii are located on the back of the upper arm and are responsible for elbow extension, which is crucial for locking out the bench press.

To perform the banded bench press, start by securing a resistance band to the base of a sturdy bench or power rack. Lay on the bench with the band positioned across your chest and grasp the band with your hands slightly wider than shoulder-width apart.

Unrack the bar and lower it to your chest, keeping your elbows tucked at a 45-degree angle to your body. As you lower the bar, the resistance from the band will increase, making the bottom portion of the lift more challenging.

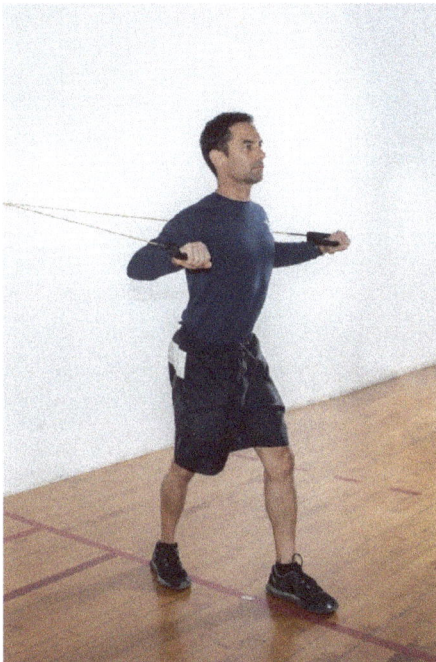

As you press the bar back up, the resistance from the band will decrease, allowing you to accelerate through the top portion of the lift. This accommodating resistance can help improve your explosiveness and power, leading to greater strength gains over time.

In addition to providing accommodating resistance, the banded bench press also challenges your stability and control. As you press the bar up, the band will try to pull it back down, forcing your muscles to work harder to maintain proper form and technique. This increased stability challenge can help improve your overall bench press performance and reduce your risk of injury.

When performing the banded bench press, it is important to maintain correct posture. Keep your feet flat on the floor, your glutes and core engaged, and your shoulder blades retracted throughout the movement. Avoid bouncing the bar off your chest or using an excessive arch in your lower back, as this can reduce the effectiveness of the exercise and increase your risk of injury.

As with any new exercise, start with a lighter resistance band and focus on perfecting your form before adding more tension. As you become more comfortable with the movement, gradually increase the resistance to continue challenging your muscles and driving progress.

Incorporating the banded bench press into your powerlifting routine can be a powerful tool for building strength, improving power, and enhancing overall performance. Whether you use it as a primary bench press variation or as an accessory movement to complement your traditional barbell bench press, the unique challenges provided by the bands can help take your training to the next level.

Variations (e.g., incline bench press, close-grip bench press)

Just like with squats, incorporating variations of the bench press can help target specific muscle groups, address weaknesses, and add variety to your training. Two common variations that can be enhanced with the use of resistance bands are the incline bench press and the close-grip bench press.

The incline bench press targets the upper chest and front shoulders more than the traditional flat bench press. To perform the banded incline bench press, set up a bench at a 30–45-degree incline and secure a resistance band to the base of the bench. Lay on the bench with the band positioned across your upper chest and grasp the band with your hands slightly wider than shoulder-width apart.

Lower the bar to your upper chest, keeping your elbows tucked at a 45-degree angle to your body. As you press the bar back up, focus on squeezing your upper chest and front shoulders to drive the movement.

The added resistance from the band will make the top portion of the lift more challenging, helping to improve your lockout strength and overall power in the incline bench press.

The close-grip bench press, on the other hand, places greater emphasis on the triceps and can be a valuable accessory movement for lifters looking to improve their lockout strength in the traditional bench press. To perform the banded close-grip bench press, set up as you would for a traditional banded bench press, but position your hands closer together, with your index fingers about shoulder-width apart.

As you lower the bar to your chest, keep your elbows tucked close to your body to emphasize the triceps. Press the bar back up, focusing on extending your elbows and squeezing your triceps at the top of the movement.

The added resistance from the band will make the top portion of the lift more challenging, helping to build strength and hypertrophy in your triceps.

When performing these bench press variations with resistance bands, start with a lighter tension and focus on maintaining proper form before progressing to heavier bands. As with any exercise, gradually increase the resistance over time to continue challenging your muscles and driving progress.

Incorporating the incline bench press and close-grip bench press with resistance bands into your powerlifting routine can help target specific muscle groups, address weaknesses, and improve overall performance. By adding variety to your training and challenging your muscles in new ways, you can continue to make progress and reach your strength and hypertrophy goals.

Overhead Press

The overhead press, also known as the military press, is a compound upper body exercise that targets the shoulders, triceps, and upper chest. While not one of the three primary lifts in powerlifting, the overhead press can be a valuable accessory movement for building overall upper body strength and improving performance in other lifts.

The primary muscles targeted during the overhead press are the deltoids (shoulders), triceps brachii (back of the upper arm), and upper pectoralis major (upper chest). The deltoids are the rounded muscles that make up the bulk of the shoulder and are responsible for shoulder flexion (raising the arm in front of the body) and abduction (raising the arm out to the side). The triceps brachii, as mentioned earlier, are located on the back of the upper arm and are responsible for elbow extension. The upper pectoralis major assists in shoulder flexion and adduction (bringing the arm across the body).

To perform the overhead press with resistance bands, start by securing a band to a sturdy anchor point at about shoulder height. Grasp the band with your hands slightly wider than shoulder-width apart and step back to create tension in the band.

Stand with your feet shoulder-width apart and your core engaged. Press the band overhead, keeping your elbows tucked close to your body as you extend your arms. As you press the band up, the resistance will increase, making the top portion of the lift more challenging.

Lower the band back down to shoulder height with control, resisting the pull of the band as you descend. Repeat for the desired number of repetitions.

When performing the overhead press with resistance bands, it is important to maintain good solid technique to maximize the effectiveness of the exercise and reduce the risk of injury. Keep your core engaged and your glutes tight throughout the movement to provide a stable base and avoid arching your lower back.

Focus on pressing the band straight up overhead, avoiding the temptation to lean back or use momentum to aid the lift. Keep your elbows tucked close to your body as you press to maximize shoulder engagement and minimize stress on the joints.

As with any exercise, start with a lighter resistance band and focus on perfecting your form before progressing to heavier tensions. Gradually increase the resistance over time to continue challenging your muscles and driving progress.

Incorporating the overhead press with resistance bands into your powerlifting routine can help build overall upper body strength, improve shoulder stability, and enhance performance in other lifts. While not a primary powerlifting movement, the overhead press can be a valuable accessory exercise for lifters looking to maximize their strength and hypertrophy gains.

Banded Overhead Press

The banded overhead press is a variation of the traditional overhead press that incorporates resistance bands to add accommodating resistance to the movement. By using bands, you can increase the difficulty of the exercise at the top of the lift, where you are typically strongest, leading to greater strength gains and improved performance.

To perform the banded overhead press, start by securing a resistance band to a sturdy anchor point at about shoulder height. Grasp the band with your hands slightly wider than shoulder-width apart and step back to create tension in the band.

Stand with your feet shoulder-width apart and your core engaged. Press the band overhead, keeping your elbows tucked close to your body as you extend your arms. As you press the band up, the resistance will increase, making the top portion of the lift more challenging.

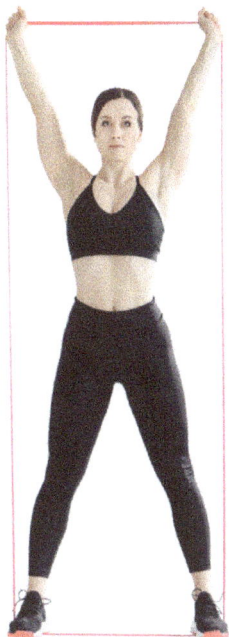

Lower the band back down to shoulder height with control, resisting the pull of the band as you descend. Repeat for the desired number of repetitions.

One of the primary benefits of the banded overhead press is the accommodating resistance provided by the bands. As you press the band overhead, the resistance increases, making the top portion of the lift more challenging. This increased tension at the top of the movement can help improve your lockout strength and power, leading to greater gains in the traditional overhead press.

In addition to providing accommodating resistance, the banded overhead press also challenges your stability and control. As you press the band overhead, it will try to pull your hands out to the sides, engaging your stabilizing muscles to keep the band in proper alignment. This increased stability challenge can help improve posture.

Chapter 5: Resistance Bands as Your Powerlifting Routine

Warm-Up Exercises with Resistance Bands

Before diving into the intense world of powerlifting with resistance bands, it is crucial to properly warm up your muscles to prevent injuries and maximize performance. Warm-up exercises with resistance bands can help activate key muscles and prepare your body for the heavy lifting ahead.

One effective warm-up exercise with resistance bands is the band pull-apart. This exercise targets the muscles in your upper back and shoulders, helping to improve posture and shoulder stability. To perform the band pull-apart, stand with your feet shoulder-width apart and hold a resistance band in front of you at chest level. Keeping your arms straight, pull the band apart by squeezing your shoulder blades together. Slowly return to the starting position and repeat for 10-15 reps.

Another beneficial warm-up exercise is the banded hip thrust. This exercise targets the glutes and hamstrings, which are essential for powerlifting movements like squats and deadlifts. To perform the banded hip thrust, place a resistance band just above your knees and lie on your back with your feet flat on the ground. Push through your heels to lift your hips towards the ceiling, squeezing your glutes at the top. Lower back down and repeat for 10-15 reps.

Incorporating these warm-up exercises with resistance bands into your powerlifting routine can help improve your performance and reduce the risk of injury. Remember to focus on proper form and technique to get the most out of your warm-up. Stay tuned for more powerlifting techniques with resistance bands to take your strength and power to the next level.

Strength Training Workouts with Resistance Bands

Strength training workouts with resistance bands are an effective way to build muscle and increase overall strength. Whether you are a beginner or a seasoned powerlifter, incorporating resistance bands into your workouts can take your training to the next level.

One of the key benefits of using resistance bands is the ability to target specific muscle groups with precision. By varying the resistance level of the bands, you can customize your workouts to match your current fitness level and goals. This makes resistance bands a versatile tool for anyone looking to improve their strength and power.

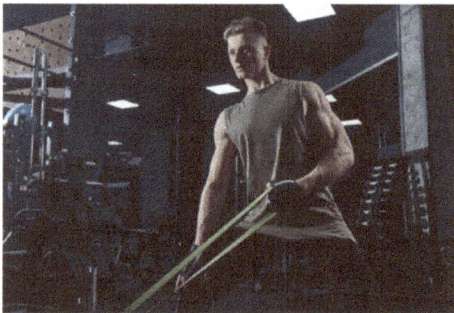

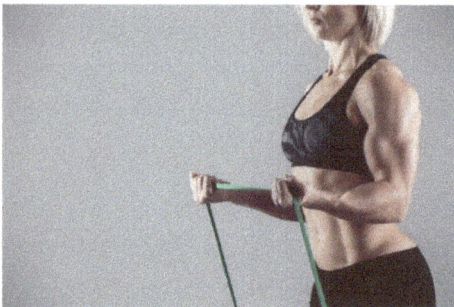

When it comes to powerlifting with resistance bands, there are a few key exercises that can help you develop the strength and muscle mass needed to excel in the sport. These exercises include squats, deadlifts, bench presses, and overhead presses, all of which can be enhanced with the use of resistance bands.

To perform a squat with resistance bands, simply place the band under your feet and hold onto the handles as you squat down. The resistance provided by the bands will help you engage your leg muscles more effectively, leading to greater gains in strength and power.

Similarly, using resistance bands during deadlifts can help you improve your grip strength and overall stability, making it easier to lift heavier weights over time. By incorporating resistance bands into your powerlifting workouts, you can challenge your muscles in new ways and push past plateaus in your training.

Overall, strength training workouts with resistance bands are a valuable addition to any powerlifting routine. Whether you are looking to increase your muscle mass, improve your strength, or enhance your powerlifting performance, resistance bands can help you achieve your goals and take your training to the next level.

Cool Down and Recovery Techniques with Resistance Bands

After a challenging powerlifting session with resistance bands, it is essential to incorporate proper cool down and recovery techniques to help your muscles recover and prevent injury. Resistance bands can be a valuable tool in aiding your body's recovery process and ensuring you are ready for your next workout.

One effective cool down technique is using resistance bands for stretching exercises. The bands can help you achieve a deeper stretch and improve flexibility in your muscles. Try incorporating resistance band stretches for your hamstrings, quadriceps, shoulders, and back to target all major muscle groups used during powerlifting.

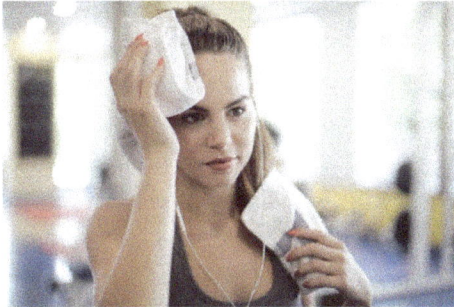

Foam rolling is another excellent recovery technique that can be enhanced with the use of resistance bands. Roll out your muscles with a foam roller while incorporating resistance bands to add extra pressure and target specific areas of tightness. This can help release muscle tension and improve blood flow to aid in recovery.

Incorporating resistance band exercises into your cool down routine can also help improve your overall strength and stability. Focus on exercises that target smaller muscle groups that may not have been activated during your powerlifting session. This can help prevent muscle imbalances and improve your overall performance in future workouts.

Remember to listen to your body during your cool down and recovery routines. If you experience any pain or discomfort, stop immediately and consult with a healthcare professional. By incorporating these cool down and recovery techniques with resistance bands into your powerlifting routine, you can optimize your performance and ensure you are ready to tackle your next workout with confidence.

Sample Workouts and Programs

In this subchapter, we will dive into some sample workouts and programs that you can follow to enhance your powerlifting techniques using resistance bands. Whether you are a beginner looking to build strength or an experienced lifter wanting to take your training to the next level, these workouts and programs will help you achieve your fitness goals.

Sample Workout 1: Full Body Strength Training This workout is perfect for those looking to improve their overall strength using resistance bands.

Perform each exercise for 3 sets of 10-12 reps.

1. Squats with Resistance Bands: 3 sets of 12 reps

2. Push-ups with Resistance Bands: 3 sets of 12 reps

3. Bent-over Rows with Resistance Bands: 3 sets of 12 reps

4. Deadlifts with Resistance Bands: 3 sets of 12 reps

5. Plank with Resistance Bands: 3 sets of 30 seconds

Sample Workout 2: Powerlifting Program
For those interested in powerlifting, this program will help you build strength and improve your technique using resistance bands. Perform each exercise for 5 sets of 5 reps.

1. **Squats with Resistance Bands**

2. **Bench Press with Resistance Bands**

3. **Deadlifts with Resistance Bands**

These sample workouts and programs are just a starting point. Feel free to customize them based on your fitness level and goals. Remember to always warm up before starting your workout and cool down afterwards to prevent injury.

With dedication and consistency, you will see improvements in your strength and powerlifting techniques by incorporating resistance bands into your training routine. Stay motivated and keep pushing yourself to reach new heights in your fitness journey.

Beginner program

The beginner program outlined in this chapter is designed to introduce individuals of all ages to the fundamentals of powerlifting with resistance bands. Whether you are a teenager looking to build strength or an older adult seeking to improve your overall fitness, this program is tailored to help you achieve your goals.

The program starts with basic movements such as squats, deadlifts, and bench press, which are essential for building a solid foundation in powerlifting. It is important to focus on ideal body placement during these exercises to prevent injury and maximize results.

As you progress through the program, you will gradually increase the resistance levels of the bands to challenge your muscles and continue to see improvements in strength and power. The program also includes variations of the main lifts to target different muscle groups and keep your workouts exciting and engaging.

In addition to the exercises, the beginner program also emphasizes the importance of proper nutrition and rest to support your training efforts. Fueling your body with the right nutrients and allowing it to recover between workouts are crucial components of a successful powerlifting program.

By following the guidelines outlined in this chapter, you will be well on your way to becoming a stronger and more powerful version of yourself. Remember, consistency is key, so stay dedicated to your training and watch as your strength and power levels soar to new heights.

Intermediate program

The intermediate program in powerlifting with resistance bands is designed to take your strength and power to the next level. This program is perfect for individuals who have some experience with powerlifting and are looking to increase their strength, improve their technique, and see some serious gains.

In this program, you will continue to focus on the three main powerlifting lifts: squat, bench press, and deadlift. However, the intensity and volume of your workouts will increase to challenge your muscles and push you to new limits. You will also be introduced to more advanced techniques and variations of the lifts to help you build muscle and improve your overall performance.

One key aspect of the intermediate program is the incorporation of resistance bands into your training routine. Resistance bands provide constant tension throughout the entire range of motion, helping you build strength and power more effectively. They also help improve your stability and balance, which are crucial for powerlifting.

In addition to the main lifts, the intermediate program will include accessory exercises to target specific muscle groups and improve your overall strength. These exercises will help you address any weaknesses or imbalances you may

110

have, improving your performance in the main lifts.

Overall, the intermediate program in powerlifting with resistance bands will challenge you both mentally and physically. It will push you to work harder, lift heavier, and become a stronger, more powerful athlete. So, if you are ready to take your powerlifting game to the next level, this program is for you.

Advanced program

Welcome to the advanced program section of "Strength and Power: Powerlifting Techniques with Resistance Bands." This subchapter is designed for those who have mastered the basics of powerlifting with resistance bands and are ready to take their training to the next level. Whether you are a teenager just starting out or a seasoned lifter looking to improve your strength and power, this program will challenge you and help you reach new heights in your powerlifting journey.

In this section, we will focus on more advanced powerlifting techniques and exercises that will push your limits and help you achieve your fitness goals. We will also introduce more complex resistance band exercises that will target specific muscle groups and improve your overall strength and power.

One of the key components of the advanced program is periodization, which involves varying your training intensity and volume over time to prevent plateaus and continue making progress. We will provide you with a structured program that includes different training phases to help you build strength, increase power, and maximize your performance on the platform.

Additionally, we will discuss advanced techniques such as accommodating resistance, dynamic effort training, and deloading to help you optimize your training and achieve peak performance. These techniques are essential for powerlifters looking to take their training to the next level and reach their full potential.

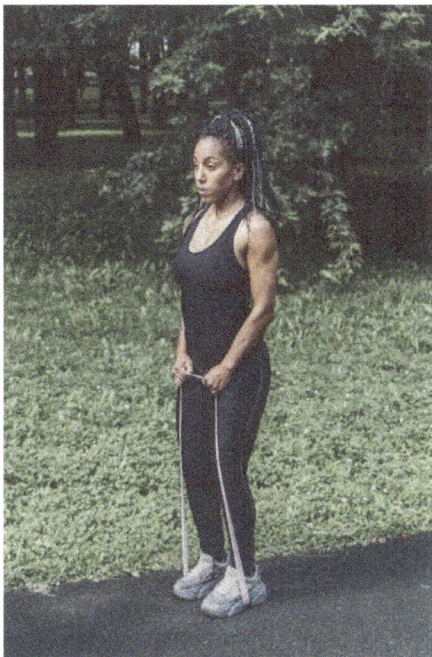

Whether you are a competitive powerlifter or simply looking to improve your strength and power, the advanced program in "Strength and Power: Powerlifting Techniques with Resistance Bands" will help you become a stronger, more powerful lifter. Get ready to challenge yourself, push your limits, and see the results you have been working towards.

The one-repetition maximum (1RM) is the heaviest weight an individual can lift for a single repetition with proper form. It is a commonly used measure of maximal strength in powerlifting and other strength-based sports. Determining your 1RM is important for setting training goals, assessing progress, and designing effective strength training programs.

Traditionally, 1RM testing is done with free weights, such as barbells and dumbbells. However, resistance bands can also be used to estimate 1RM, offering a safer and more accessible alternative to heavy weights. In this article, we will explore the differences between

1RM testing with bands and weights and provide guidelines for performing a 1RM test using resistance bands.

1RM Testing with Weights

When testing 1RM with weights, the goal is to find the heaviest load you can lift for a single repetition while maintaining form. This process typically involves gradually increasing the weight until you reach your maximum capacity. Here is a step-by-step guide to performing a 1RM test with weights:

1. Warm-up: Begin with a general warm-up to increase blood flow and prepare your muscles for the upcoming effort. Perform 5-10 minutes of light cardio followed by dynamic stretching.

2. Specific warm-up: Perform a specific warm-up using the exercise you will be testing. Start with

a light weight and perform 5-10 repetitions. Rest for 1-2 minutes.

3. Increase the weight: Add weight to the bar and perform 3-5 repetitions. The weight should be challenging but not close to your maximum. Rest for 2-3 minutes.

4. Increase weight again: Add more weight and perform 2-3 repetitions. This weight should be close to your estimated 1RM. Rest for 3-4 minutes.

5. 1RM attempts: Increase the weight to your estimated 1RM and attempt a single repetition. If successful, rest for 3-5 minutes and increase your weight for your next attempt. If unsuccessful, rest for 3-5 minutes and decrease the weight slightly for your next attempt.

6. Continue 1RM attempts: Keep increasing or decreasing the weight as necessary until you find the heaviest weight you can lift for a single repetition with proper form.

It is important to note that 1RM testing with weights can be physically and mentally demanding. It requires proper technique, safety precautions, and the presence of a spotter. Individuals should have a solid foundation of strength training experience before attempting a 1RM test with weights.

1RM Testing with Resistance Bands

Testing 1RM with resistance bands is a safer and more accessible alternative to using heavy weights. Resistance bands provide accommodating resistance, meaning the resistance increases as the band stretches. This unique property allows for a challenging stimulus without the need for heavy loads. Here is how to perform a 1RM test using resistance bands:

1. Warm-up: Follow the same general warm-up protocol as described for testing with weights.

117

2. Select the appropriate band: Choose a resistance band that provides enough tension to challenge you for a single repetition. This may require some trial and error.

3. Specific warm-up: Perform a specific warm-up using the exercise you will be testing with the selected band. Perform 5-10 repetitions. Rest for 1-2 minutes.

4. Increase the tension: If the initial band was too easy, select a band with greater resistance. If the band was too challenging, select a lighter band. Perform 2-3 repetitions with the new band. Rest for 2-3 minutes.

5. 1RM attempts: Perform a single repetition with the selected band. If successful, rest for 2-3 minutes and select a band with greater resistance for your next attempt. If unsuccessful, rest for 2-3 minutes and select a lighter band for your next attempt.

6. Continue 1RM attempts: Keep adjusting the band resistance as necessary until you find the band that allows you to perform a single repetition with proper form.

When testing 1RM with resistance bands, it is important to maintain proper form and control throughout the movement. Focus on a smooth, deliberate tempo and avoid using momentum or compromising your technique. It may be helpful to have a partner assist you in selecting the appropriate band and providing feedback on your form.

Advantages of 1RM Testing with Resistance Bands

Testing 1RM with resistance bands offers several advantages compared to traditional weight-based testing:

1. Safety: Resistance bands provide a safer alternative to heavy weights, reducing the risk of injury during maximal attempts. If you lose control of the band, it will not cause the same level of harm as dropping a heavy barbell.

2. Accessibility: Resistance bands are portable, affordable, and easy to use in various settings. They allow for 1RM testing at home, in a hotel room, or outdoors without the need for expensive equipment or a gym membership.

3. Accommodating resistance: The increasing tension provided by resistance bands challenges your muscles throughout the entire range of motion. This unique stimulus can lead to greater strength gains and muscle activation compared to traditional free weights.

4. Versatility: Resistance bands can be used to test 1RM for a wide variety of exercises, including upper body, lower body, and core movements. They allow for greater flexibility in exercise selection compared to weight-based testing.

5. Reduced joint stress: The accommodating resistance of bands places less stress on the joints compared to heavy weights. This can be particularly beneficial for individuals with joint issues or those recovering from injury.

Limitations of 1RM Testing with Resistance Bands

While 1RM testing with resistance bands offers several advantages, there are also some limitations to consider:

1. Difficulty in quantifying resistance: Unlike free weights, resistance bands do not have a standardized system for quantifying resistance. The tension provided by a band can vary based on its length, thickness, and material. This makes it challenging to accurately compare 1RM values between individuals or track progress over time.

2. Limited maximal resistance: While resistance bands can provide a challenging stimulus, they may not offer enough resistance for advanced lifters or those with high levels of maximal strength. In these cases, traditional weight-based testing may be necessary to accurately assess 1RM.

3. Technique differences: The technique used for exercises with resistance bands may differ slightly from their free weight counterparts. This can make it challenging to directly compare 1RM values between band-based and weight-based testing.

4. Stability challenges: Resistance bands can be unstable, particularly at elevated levels of tension. This instability can make it difficult to maintain proper form and control during maximal attempts, potentially increasing the risk of injury.

Conclusion

One-repetition maximum (1RM) testing is a valuable tool for assessing maximal strength and designing effective strength training programs. While traditionally performed with free weights, 1RM testing can also be done using resistance bands. Band-based testing offers a safer, more accessible, and versatile alternative to heavy weights, making it a useful option for a wide range of individuals.

When testing 1RM with resistance bands, it is important to follow proper warm-up protocols, select an appropriate level of resistance, and maintain proper form and control throughout the movement. While there are some limitations to band-based testing, such as difficulty in quantifying resistance and limited maximal resistance, the advantages of safety, accessibility, accommodating resistance, versatility, and reduced joint stress make it a valuable tool for many lifters.

The choice between band-based and weight-based 1RM testing will depend on individual goals, experience level, and access to equipment. By understanding the differences between these two methods and their respective advantages and limitations, individuals can make an informed decision on which approach best suits their needs. Regardless of the method chosen, regularly assessing 1RM can provide valuable insights into an individual's strength levels and help guide the design of effective training programs for continued progress and performance enhancement.

Chapter 6: Advanced Powerlifting Strategies with Resistance Bands

Progressive Overload with Resistance Bands

Progressive overload, a fundamental principle in strength training, involves gradually increasing the demands placed on the muscles over time. This concept is crucial for achieving continuous improvements in strength and power. When it comes to powerlifting with resistance bands, progressive overload is essential for maximizing gains and reaching full potential.

Resistance bands, known for their versatility, can be easily adjusted to provide varying levels of resistance, making them an ideal tool for implementing progressive overload into powerlifting routines. By gradually increasing the resistance of the bands as strength improves, lifters can ensure that their muscles are constantly challenged, forcing them to adapt and grow.

One effective method to implement progressive overload with resistance bands is to increase the tension by using thicker bands or doubling up on bands. This increased resistance will make exercises more challenging, requiring muscles to work harder to overcome the added tension. Another approach is to increase the number of sets and repetitions performed with the bands, further challenging the muscles, and promoting growth.

It is crucial to remember that progressive overload should be implemented gradually and safely to reduce the risk of injury. Lifters must listen to their bodies and pay attention to how they respond to the increased resistance. If any pain or discomfort is experienced, it is important to reduce the intensity and reassess the approach.

When incorporating progressive overload with resistance bands into a powerlifting routine, it is essential to focus on the primary lifts: squats, bench press, and deadlifts. For squats, lifters can use bands to add resistance at the top of the movement, challenging the quadriceps and glutes. In the bench press, bands can be used to increase tension at the lockout position, targeting the triceps and chest muscles. For deadlifts, bands can be used to provide resistance throughout the entire range of motion, engaging the posterior chain muscles, including the hamstrings, glutes, and lower back.

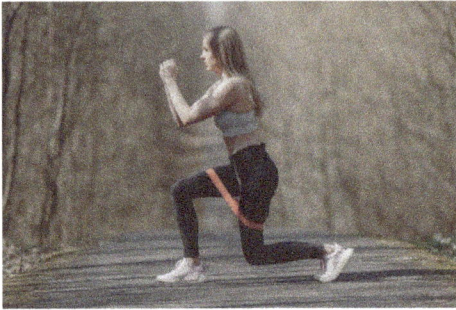

In addition to the primary lifts, resistance bands can be used to progressively overload accessory exercises. For example, banded push-ups can be used to target the chest and triceps, while banded rows can be used to target the back and biceps. By increasing the resistance of the bands used in these exercises over time, lifters can continue to challenge their muscles and promote growth.

Progressive overload with resistance bands can also be used to target specific weak points in a lifter's technique or strength. For example, if a lifter struggles with lockout strength in the bench press, they can use bands to provide increased resistance at the top of the movement, helping to strengthen this specific area.

To effectively implement progressive overload with resistance bands, it is important to keep track of the resistance used and the number of sets and repetitions performed. This can be done using a training log or a spreadsheet, allowing lifters to monitor their progress over time and adjust as needed.

In addition to the physical benefits of progressive overload with resistance bands, this approach can also provide mental benefits. By consistently challenging the body and seeing progress over time, lifters can build confidence and motivation, which can translate to improved performance in the gym and on the platform.

Incorporating progressive overload with resistance bands into a powerlifting routine can be a game-changer for those looking to take their strength and power to the next level. By gradually increasing the resistance of the bands and challenging the muscles in new ways, lifters can achieve continuous gains and reach their full potential. However, it is crucial to approach progressive overload with caution, listening to the body and adjusting as needed to prevent injury and ensure long-term success in the sport of powerlifting.

Deloading and Tapering with Resistance Bands

Deloading and tapering are critical components of any well-rounded strength training program, including powerlifting with resistance bands. Deloading refers to a planned reduction in training intensity and volume to facilitate recovery and prevent overtraining, while tapering involves a gradual decrease in training volume and intensity leading up to a competition or peak performance phase.

When incorporating resistance bands into a powerlifting training program, deloading and tapering can be effectively implemented to optimize performance and minimize the risk of burnout. Deloading with resistance bands involves reducing the number of sets and repetitions performed, as well as using lighter resistance bands to allow the muscles to recover from heavy loads. This strategic approach helps prevent injuries and ensures that the body is fully recovered before progressing to more intense training phases.

Tapering with resistance bands is crucial for achieving peak performance during competitions. By gradually reducing training volume and intensity while still incorporating resistance bands, lifters can maintain strength and power while providing their bodies with the necessary rest to perform optimally on competition day. Tapering also helps minimize fatigue and ensures that lifters are fresh and prepared to achieve new personal records.

When implementing deloading and tapering strategies with resistance bands, it is essential to consider the individual needs and goals of each lifter. Factors such as training experience, recovery ability, and competition schedule should be considered when designing a deloading and tapering plan.

For novice lifters, deloading with resistance bands may involve a more significant reduction in training volume and intensity, as their bodies may require more time to adapt to the demands of powerlifting. On the other hand, experienced lifters may be able to handle a more gradual reduction in volume and intensity during a deload phase.

When it comes to tapering with resistance bands, the duration and intensity of the taper will depend on the length and importance of the competition. For a major competition, lifters may begin tapering 2-3 weeks in advance, gradually reducing volume and intensity each week while maintaining the use of resistance bands to prevent detraining.

During a deload or taper phase, it is important to focus on maintaining proper form and technique with resistance bands. This is an excellent opportunity to work on refining movement patterns and addressing any technical inefficiencies without the added stress of heavy loads.

In addition to reducing training volume and intensity, deloading and tapering with resistance bands should also involve a focus on recovery modalities. This may include techniques such as foam rolling, stretching, and massage to promote muscle relaxation and reduce the risk of injury.

Nutrition also plays a crucial role in the success of deloading and tapering with resistance bands. During these phases, lifters should focus on consuming a balanced diet that provides adequate protein, carbohydrates, and healthy fats to support recovery and maintain muscle mass.

Incorporating deloading and tapering strategies with resistance bands into a powerlifting routine is essential for long-term success and injury prevention. By listening to the body, adjusting training volume and intensity, and utilizing resistance bands effectively, lifters can optimize their performance and achieve their powerlifting goals.

It is important to remember that deloading and tapering are highly individualized processes, and what works for one lifter may not work for another. Lifters should work closely with a qualified coach or trainer to develop a deloading and tapering plan that is tailored to their specific needs and goals.

By prioritizing recovery and incorporating deloading and tapering with resistance bands into a powerlifting program, lifters can avoid plateaus, minimize the risk of injury, and achieve peak performance when it matters most. With a strategic approach to training and recovery, lifters can unlock their full potential and enjoy long-term success in the sport of powerlifting.

Peak Performance Strategies for Powerlifting Competitions

Powerlifting competitions require a combination of physical and mental preparation to achieve peak performance. Implementing the right strategies, including the use of resistance bands, can make a significant difference in a lifter's success on the platform. This subchapter will explore key peak performance strategies that can help powerlifters excel in competitions while utilizing resistance bands.

Mental preparation is a critical component of peak performance in powerlifting. Visualizing success, setting specific goals, and maintaining focus on performance can help lifters stay motivated and confident throughout the competition. Incorporating techniques such as positive self-talk and mindfulness can help lifters maintain a positive mindset and perform at their best.

In addition to mental preparation, physical preparation is essential for peak performance in powerlifting competitions. This includes following a well-designed training program that incorporates resistance bands to develop strength, refine technique, and reduce the risk of injury. Lifters should focus on developing power, speed, and explosiveness in their lifts to maximize performance on competition day.

When using resistance bands in preparation for a competition, lifters should focus on exercises that target the primary lifts: squats, bench press, and deadlifts. For squats, resistance bands can be used to provide accommodating resistance, challenging the muscles throughout the entire range of motion. This can help lifters develop power out of the hole and improve their ability to stand up with heavy loads.

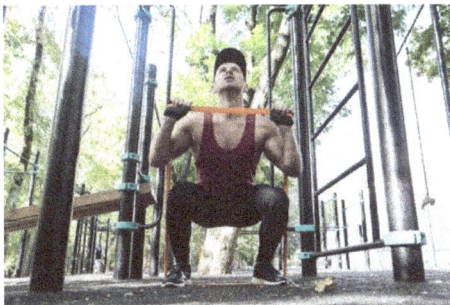

For bench press, resistance bands can be used to increase tension at the lockout position, helping lifters develop the strength and power needed to complete the lift. Bands can also be used to work on speed and explosiveness off the chest, a critical component of a successful bench press.

In the deadlift, resistance bands can be used to provide resistance throughout the entire range of motion, engaging the posterior chain muscles and helping lifters develop the strength and power needed to pull heavy loads off the floor.

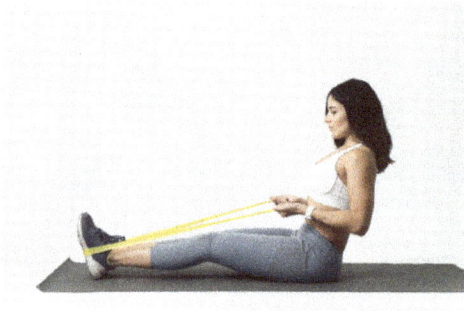

In addition to the primary lifts, resistance bands can be used to target specific weaknesses or areas of improvement. For example, if a lifter struggles with upper back strength in the squat, they can incorporate banded good mornings or banded rows into their training program to address this weakness.

Proper nutrition and hydration are also critical for peak performance in powerlifting competitions. Lifters should focus on consuming a balanced diet that provides adequate protein, carbohydrates, and healthy fats to support training and competition goals. Staying hydrated is also essential for maintaining energy levels and optimizing performance during the competition.

Rest and recovery are equally important for peak performance in powerlifting competitions. Lifters should prioritize sleep, manage stress, and incorporate active recovery techniques to stay fresh, focused, and ready to perform at their best on competition day.

When it comes to the competition itself, lifters should have a clear plan in place for warm-ups, attempts, and rest periods between lifts. Resistance bands can be used during warm-ups to help lifters prepare their muscles and joints for the demands of heavy lifting.

During the competition, lifters should focus on executing each lift with correct execution, trusting in the training they have done leading up to the event. Mental strategies such as visualization and positive self-talk can be used to stay focused and motivated throughout the competition.

After the competition, lifters should take time to reflect on their performance, identifying areas of strength and areas for improvement. This reflection can be used to inform future training cycles and peak performance strategies.

By implementing these peak performance strategies and utilizing resistance bands in training, powerlifters can improve their performance and achieve their goals in competition. Consistency, dedication, and a positive mindset are key to success in powerlifting with resistance bands.

In conclusion, peak performance in powerlifting competitions requires a comprehensive approach that includes mental preparation, physical training with resistance bands, proper nutrition and hydration, rest and recovery, and a clear competition plan. By focusing on these key strategies and utilizing the unique benefits of resistance bands, lifters can unlock their full potential and achieve success on the platform.

Chapter 7: Common Mistakes to Avoid in Powerlifting with Resistance Bands

Using Incorrect Form with Resistance Bands

Incorporating resistance bands into your powerlifting routine can be an effective way to improve strength and power, but using incorrect form can lead to suboptimal results and increase the risk of injury. It is crucial to understand and execute proper techniques when utilizing resistance bands in your training.

One of the most common mistakes made when using resistance bands is employing too much resistance. While it may be tempting to select the thickest band available, doing so can cause you to compromise your form to complete the exercise. This not only diminishes the effectiveness of the workout but also places undue stress on your muscles and joints. To avoid this pitfall, begin with a resistance level that allows you to maintain proper form throughout the entire range of motion.

Another frequent error is using improper alignment when performing exercises with resistance bands. This can manifest in several ways, such as rounding your back, arching your spine, or allowing your knees to collapse inward. These misalignments can increase the risk of injury and prevent you from effectively targeting the intended muscle groups. To ensure optimal results and safety, pay close attention to your body positioning and make necessary adjustments to maintain proper alignment.

Rushing through exercises with resistance bands is another mistake that can lead to improper form and diminish the efficacy of your workout. It is essential to focus on controlled movements and precise technique to guarantee that you are targeting the correct muscles and maximizing the benefits of your training. Take the time to execute each repetition with intention and control, rather than prioritizing speed or quantity.

When using resistance bands for specific powerlifting movements, such as squats, deadlifts, and bench presses, it is critical to maintain proper form to avoid injury and ensure that you are effectively targeting the intended muscle groups. For squats, keep your chest up, core engaged, and knees in line with your toes. When performing deadlifts, maintain a neutral spine, engage your lasts, and drive through your heels. For bench presses, keep your shoulders retracted, elbows tucked, and feet firmly planted on the ground.

In addition to these general form considerations, it is important to be mindful of the unique challenges presented by resistance bands. Unlike traditional free weights, resistance bands provide variable resistance throughout the range of motion, with the tension increasing as the band stretches. This means that the resistance will be greatest at the top of the movement, which can be challenging for some lifters. To accommodate for this, focus on maintaining tension throughout the entire range of motion and avoid relaxing at the top of the movement.

Another consideration when using resistance bands is the potential for the bands to slip or roll during the exercise. To prevent this, ensure that the bands are securely anchored and that you are using a stable surface to stand on. If you are using bands with handles, make sure that your grip is secure and that the handles are not slipping in your hands.

145

To further optimize your form when using resistance bands, consider incorporating accessory exercises that target specific muscle groups and help to reinforce proper technique. For example, banded glute bridges can help to strengthen the glutes and improve hip extension, which is crucial for squats and deadlifts. Banded face pulls can help to strengthen the upper back and improve posture, which is important for bench presses and overhead presses.

By paying attention to your form and technique when using resistance bands, you can maximize the benefits of your powerlifting routine while minimizing the risk of injury. Take the time to learn and practice proper techniques and be willing to adjust as needed to ensure that you are getting the most out of your workouts. With consistent effort and attention to detail, you can achieve your powerlifting goals and avoid the common mistakes associated with using resistance bands.

Overtraining with Resistance Bands

Overtraining is a common pitfall that many powerlifters encounter when incorporating resistance bands into their training regimen. While resistance bands can be a highly effective tool for increasing strength and power, it is crucial to use them judiciously to prevent overtraining and its associated negative consequences.

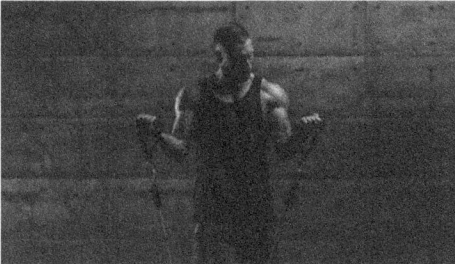

Overtraining occurs when an individual pushes their body beyond its capacity to recover, leading to a host of physiological and psychological symptoms. These can include decreased performance, increased fatigue, muscle soreness, irritability, and even injury. When using resistance bands, it can be tempting to constantly increase the resistance or volume of training to make rapid progress. However, this approach can quickly lead to overtraining if not carefully managed.

One of the key factors contributing to overtraining with resistance bands is a lack of proper periodization. Periodization refers to the strategic planning of training cycles to optimize progress and prevent overtraining. When using resistance bands, it is important to vary the intensity, volume, and frequency of training to allow for adequate recovery and adaptation. *This may involve incorporating deload weeks, where the intensity and volume of training are reduced to allow for recovery or alternating between heavy and light training days to manage fatigue.*

Another factor that can contribute to overtraining with resistance bands is a lack of variety in training. While it may be tempting to focus solely on the "big three" powerlifting movements (squats, deadlifts, and bench presses), neglecting other muscle groups and movement patterns can lead to imbalances and overuse injuries. Incorporating a variety of exercises that target different muscle groups and planes of motion can help to prevent overtraining and promote overall physical development.

In addition to proper periodization and exercise selection, adequate nutrition and sleep are critical for preventing overtraining with resistance bands. Resistance training places significant demands on the body, and proper nutrition is necessary to support recovery and adaptation. This includes consuming adequate protein to support muscle repair and growth, as well as carbohydrates to replenish glycogen stores and support energy levels. Adequate sleep is also crucial for recovery, with most experts recommending 7-9 hours per night for optimal physical and mental performance.

Another important consideration when using resistance bands to prevent overtraining is the use of form. Using improper form or technique can place excessive stress on the joints and connective tissues, increasing the risk of injury and overtraining. When using resistance bands, it is important to focus on maintaining proper alignment, engaging the appropriate muscle groups, and controlling the movement throughout the entire range of motion.

To further reduce the risk of overtraining with resistance bands, it can be helpful to incorporate other recovery modalities into your training regimen. This may include techniques such as foam rolling, massage, and stretching to promote muscle relaxation and reduce soreness. Active recovery, such as low-intensity cardiovascular exercise or light resistance training, can also be beneficial for promoting blood flow and reducing muscle soreness.

The key to preventing overtraining with resistance bands is to listen to your body and be willing to adjust your training as needed. If you experience persistent fatigue, muscle soreness, or decreased performance, it may be a sign that you are overtraining and need to reduce the intensity or volume of your training. By being proactive and responsive to your body's needs, you can avoid the negative consequences of overtraining and continue to make progress in your powerlifting journey.

Ignoring Recovery and Rest Days

One of the most common mistakes made by powerlifters, regardless of their experience level or the equipment they use, is ignoring the importance of recovery and rest days. When training with resistance bands, it can be easy to fall into the trap of thinking that because the resistance is less than traditional free weights, you can train more frequently or with greater intensity. However, this mindset can quickly lead to overtraining, burnout, and even injury.

Recovery and rest days are essential components of any successful powerlifting program, whether you are using resistance bands or free weights. During these days, your body has the opportunity to repair and rebuild the muscle tissue that has been broken down during training. This process, known as muscle protein synthesis, is critical for increasing strength, power, and muscle mass over time.

When you ignore recovery, rest days, and continue to train with high intensity or frequency, you are short-circuiting this process. Instead of allowing your muscles to fully recover and adapt to the training stimulus, you are constantly breaking them down further, leading to a state of chronic fatigue and decreased performance.

In addition to the physiological consequences of ignoring recovery and rest days, there are also psychological factors to consider. Training with high intensity and frequency can be mentally taxing, leading to burnout, decreased motivation, and even depression. Taking regular rest days can help to prevent these negative psychological effects and maintain a positive and enthusiastic approach to training.

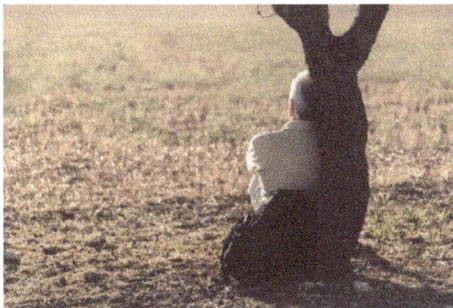

So, how can you ensure that you are incorporating adequate recovery and rest days into your powerlifting program with resistance bands? The first step is to create a structured training plan that includes a balance of high-intensity training days and low-intensity or rest days. This may involve training with resistance bands 3-4 times per week, with 1-2 days of complete rest or active recovery in between.

On your rest days, it is important to engage in activities that promote recovery and relaxation. This may include gentle stretching, foam rolling, or massage to help reduce muscle soreness and promote blood flow. Light cardiovascular exercise, such as walking or cycling, can also be beneficial for promoting recovery and maintaining cardiovascular fitness.

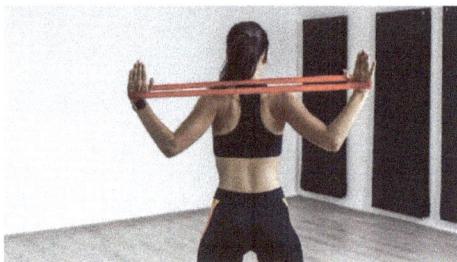

In addition to structured rest days, it is also important to listen to your body and be willing to take additional rest as needed. If you are feeling particularly fatigued, sore, or unmotivated, it may be a sign that you need an extra day of rest to allow your body to fully recover. Pushing through these feelings and continuing to train can lead to overtraining and injury.

Another important aspect of recovery when training with resistance bands proper nutrition is. Consuming adequate protein, carbohydrates, and healthy fats can help to support muscle repair and growth, as well as maintain energy levels throughout your training. Staying hydrated is also crucial for optimal performance and recovery, so be sure to drink plenty of water throughout the day.

Finally, it is important to remember that recovery and rest days are not a sign of weakness or lack of dedication. In fact, taking the time to prioritize recovery can enhance your long-term progress and performance. By allowing your body the time it needs to adapt and grow stronger, you can avoid plateaus and continue to make gains over time.

Ignoring recovery and rest days is a common mistake made by powerlifters of all levels, but it is one that can have profound consequences for your health and performance. By incorporating structured rest days, engaging in active recovery, listening to your body, and prioritizing proper nutrition and hydration, you can optimize your recovery and make consistent progress in your powerlifting journey with resistance bands.

Chapter 8: The Benefits of Resistance Band Training for Powerlifters: Saving Time, Space, and Money

In the world of powerlifting, where heavy weights and complex equipment are often seen as essential tools for success, resistance bands offer a unique and often overlooked alternative. While traditional barbell training will always have its place in the sport, incorporating resistance bands into a powerlifting routine can provide a range of benefits, particularly for lifters who are short on time, space, or financial resources.

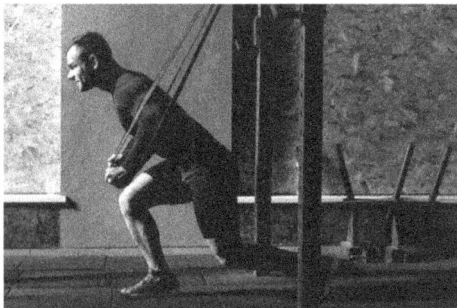

One of the most significant advantages of resistance band training for powerlifters is the ability to save space. Unlike traditional weightlifting equipment, which can take up a significant amount of room and require a dedicated training space, resistance bands are compact and easy to store. A full set of bands can easily fit into a small bag or drawer, making them an ideal option for lifters who live in small apartments, have limited storage space, or simply prefer a minimalist training setup.

This space-saving benefit of resistance bands is particularly valuable for powerlifters who train at home. With a simple set of bands and a few basic accessories, such as a door anchor or a sturdy pole, lifters can create a full-body workout routine that targets all the major muscle groups and supports their powerlifting goals. This eliminates the need for expensive and bulky equipment, such as a squat rack, bench press, or weight plates, making it possible to build strength and muscle in even the smallest of spaces.

Another key benefit of resistance band training for powerlifters is the ability to save time. Traditional barbell training often requires a significant amount of setup and breakdown time, particularly when using heavy weights or complex equipment. This can be a major drawback for lifters who have busy schedules or limited time to dedicate to their training.

With resistance bands, however, setup and breakdown time is minimal. Bands can be quickly attached to a door anchor or wrapped around a pole, allowing lifters to transition from one exercise to the next with ease. This makes it possible to complete a full-body workout in a shorter amount of time, without sacrificing the quality or intensity of the training.

Furthermore, resistance band training can be easily integrated into a busy lifestyle. Because bands are so portable and easy to use, lifters can take their workouts with them wherever they go. Whether traveling for work or pleasure, or simply looking to fit in a quick workout during a lunch break, resistance bands make it possible to maintain a consistent training routine no matter where life takes you.

In addition to saving time and space, resistance band training can also be a cost-effective option for powerlifters. Traditional weightlifting equipment, such as barbells, weight plates, and machines, can be expensive, particularly for lifters who are just starting out or who have limited financial resources. Resistance bands, on the other hand, are inexpensive, with a full set of high-quality bands costing a fraction of the price of a basic barbell set.

This cost-saving benefit of resistance bands can be particularly valuable for lifters who are working with a tight budget or who are looking to build a home gym on a limited budget. By investing in a set of bands and a few basic accessories, lifters can create a full-body workout routine that supports their powerlifting goals without breaking the bank.

Of course, it is important to note that resistance band training is not a perfect substitute for traditional barbell training. Barbells and weight plates will always have their place in powerlifting, particularly for lifters who are focused on maximizing their strength and power. However, by incorporating resistance bands into their training routines, powerlifters can enjoy a range of benefits that can support their overall goals and help them to build strength and muscle in a more efficient and cost-effective way.

When designing a resistance band training program for powerlifting, it is important to focus on exercises that target the primary muscle groups involved in the squat, bench press, and deadlift. This may include exercises such as banded squats, banded bench presses, banded deadlifts, and a variety of accessory movements that target the legs, back, chest, shoulders, and arms.

It is also important to progress the resistance over time, just as one would with traditional barbell training. As the lifter becomes stronger and more comfortable with the exercises, they can increase the resistance by using thicker bands or by combining multiple bands to create a more challenging workout.

In addition to the physical benefits of resistance band training, there are also several mental and emotional benefits that can support a powerlifter's overall well-being. Because resistance band training is so convenient and accessible, it can help to reduce the stress and anxiety that often comes with trying to fit a workout into a busy schedule. By eliminating the need to travel to a gym or spend hours setting up and breaking down equipment, lifters can focus on their training and enjoy the process of building strength and muscle.

Furthermore, resistance band training can be a wonderful way to add variety to a powerlifting routine and prevent boredom or burnout. By incorporating different exercises and resistance levels, lifters can keep their workouts fresh and engaging, even if they are limited to a small training space.

Resistance band training offers a range of benefits for powerlifters who are looking to save time, space, and money. By incorporating bands into their training routines, lifters can build strength and muscle in a convenient, cost-effective, and efficient way, without sacrificing the quality or intensity of their workouts. Whether used as a standalone training method or as a complement to traditional barbell training, resistance bands are a valuable tool that every powerlifter should consider adding to their arsenal. So, if you are a powerlifter who is short on time, space, or financial resources, give resistance band training a try – you may be surprised at just how effective it can be.

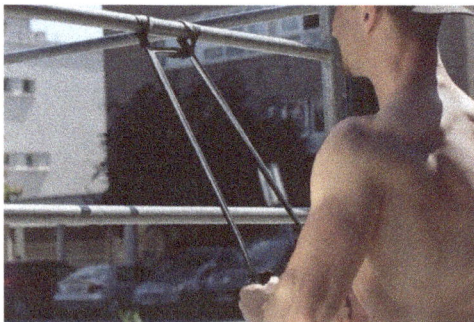

Chapter 9: Common Mistakes to Avoid in Powerlifting with Resistance Bands

Using Incorrect Form with Resistance Bands

Incorporating resistance bands into your powerlifting routine can be an incredibly effective way to improve strength, power, and overall performance. However, using incorrect form when training with resistance bands can not only lead to suboptimal results but also increase the risk of injury. To maximize the benefits of resistance band training and minimize the potential for harm, it is crucial to understand and execute proper techniques.

One of the most common mistakes made when using resistance bands is employing too much resistance. It can be tempting to select the thickest, most challenging band available to make rapid progress or push yourself to the limit. However, using a band that is too heavy can cause you to compromise your form to complete the exercise. This not only diminishes the effectiveness of the workout but also places undue stress on your muscles and joints, potentially leading to strain or injury. To avoid this pitfall, it is important to begin with a resistance level that allows you to maintain proper form throughout the entire range of motion. As you become more comfortable with the exercise and your strength improves, you can gradually

166

increase your resistance to continue challenging your muscles.

Another frequent error when training with resistance bands is using improper alignment or body positioning. This can manifest in numerous ways, such as rounding your back during deadlifts, arching your spine during squats, or allowing your knees to collapse inward during lunges or other lower body exercises. These misalignments can place excessive stress on your joints and connective tissues, increasing the risk of injury and preventing you from effectively targeting the intended muscle groups. To ensure optimal results and minimize the risk of injury, it is essential to pay close attention to your body positioning and make any necessary adjustments to maintain proper alignment. This may involve engaging your core to maintain a neutral spine, keeping your knees in line with your toes, or retracting your shoulder blades to protect your shoulders.

Rushing through exercises with resistance bands is another common mistake that can lead to improper form and diminish the efficacy of your workout. When training with resistance bands, it can be easy to get caught up in the momentum of the band and allow it to dictate the pace of your repetitions. However, this can cause you to sacrifice form and control in favor of speed or quantity. To maximize the benefits of resistance band training, it is essential to focus on controlled, deliberate movements and precise technique. Take the time to execute each repetition with intention and focus, ensuring that you are targeting the correct muscles and maintaining proper alignment throughout the entire range of motion. By prioritizing quality over quantity, you can ensure that you are getting the most out of your resistance band training and minimizing the risk of injury.

When using resistance bands for specific powerlifting movements, such as squats, deadlifts, and bench presses, it is especially critical to maintain proper form to avoid injury and ensure that you are effectively targeting the intended muscle groups. For squats, this means keeping your chest up, engaging your core to maintain a neutral spine, and ensuring that your knees remain in line with your toes throughout the movement. When performing deadlifts with resistance bands, it is important to maintain a neutral spine, engage your lats to keep the bar close to your body, and drive through your heels to activate your posterior chain. For bench presses, focus on keeping your shoulders retracted, tucking your elbows at a 45-degree angle to your body, and keeping your feet firmly planted on the ground to provide stability.

In addition to these general form considerations, it is important to be mindful of the unique challenges presented by resistance bands. Unlike traditional free weights, resistance bands provide variable resistance throughout the range of motion, with the tension increasing as the band stretches. This means that the resistance will be greatest at the top of the movement, which can be challenging for some lifters who are accustomed to the constant resistance provided by free weights. To accommodate for this

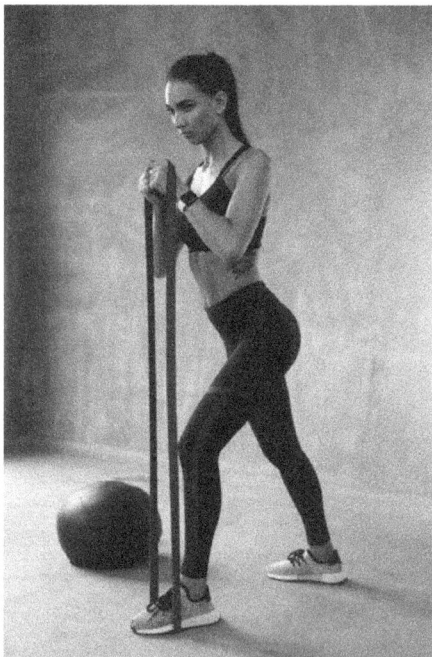

variable resistance, it is important to focus on maintaining tension throughout the entire range of motion and avoid relaxing or losing control at the top of the movement. This may require a slight adjustment to your technique or a greater emphasis on control and stability.

Another consideration when using resistance bands is the potential for the bands to slip or roll during the exercise. This can be especially problematic when using bands with handles, as the handles can rotate or slip in your hands, compromising your grip and control. To prevent this, it is important to ensure that the bands are securely anchored and that you are using a stable surface to stand on. If you are using bands with handles, make sure that your grip is secure and that you are actively engaging your forearms and hands to maintain control of the handles throughout the movement.

To further optimize your form when using resistance bands, consider incorporating accessory exercises that target specific muscle

171

groups and help to reinforce proper technique. For example, banded glute bridges can be an excellent way to strengthen the glutes and improve hip extension, which is crucial for movements like squats and deadlifts. Banded face pulls can help to strengthen the upper back and improve posture, which is important for maintaining proper alignment during bench presses and overhead presses. By incorporating these accessory exercises into your resistance band training, you can address specific weaknesses or imbalances and improve your overall form and technique.

Ultimately, the key to avoiding incorrect form when using resistance bands is to prioritize proper technique overweight or repetitions. Take the time to learn and practice the proper form for each exercise and be willing to adjust your technique or reduce the resistance as needed to maintain control and alignment. By focusing on quality over quantity and being mindful of the unique challenges presented by resistance bands, you can maximize the benefits of your resistance band training and minimize the risk of injury. With consistent effort and attention to detail, you can achieve your powerlifting goals and avoid the common mistakes associated with using resistance bands.

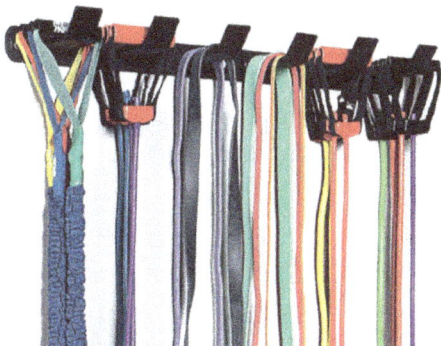

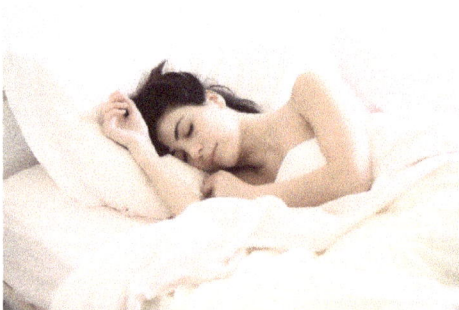

Using improper form or technique can place excessive stress on the joints, connective tissues, and muscles, increasing the risk of injury and overtraining. When using resistance bands, it is important to focus on maintaining proper alignment, engaging the appropriate muscle groups, and controlling the movement throughout the entire range of motion. If you are unsure about proper form or technique, consider working with a qualified trainer or coach who can provide guidance and feedback.

To further reduce the risk of overtraining with resistance bands, it can be helpful to incorporate other recovery modalities into your training regimen. This may include techniques such as foam rolling, massage, stretching, and active recovery. Foam rolling can help to improve circulation, reduce muscle tension, and promote relaxation. Massage can help to break up adhesions, improve flexibility, and reduce muscle soreness. Stretching can help to improve range of motion, reduce muscle tightness, and promote relaxation. Active recovery, such as low-intensity cardiovascular exercise or light resistance training, can help to promote blood flow, reduce muscle soreness, and support overall recovery.

Ultimately, the key to preventing overtraining with resistance bands is to listen to your body and be willing to adjust your training as needed. If you experience persistent fatigue, muscle soreness, or decreased performance despite adequate rest and recovery, it may be a sign that you are overtraining and need to reduce the intensity or volume of your training. By being proactive and responsive to your body's needs, you can avoid the negative consequences of overtraining and continue to make progress in your powerlifting journey.

Chapter 10: Conclusion and Next Steps

Recap of Powerlifting Techniques with Resistance Bands

Throughout this book, we have explored the various powerlifting techniques that can be effectively executed using resistance bands. These versatile training tools have proven to be a valuable asset for powerlifters of all skill levels, offering a range of benefits that can enhance strength, power, muscle activation, and overall performance.

One of the most crucial aspects of powerlifting with resistance bands is maintaining proper form and technique. This involves paying close attention to body alignment, core engagement, and controlled movement patterns. By focusing on these key elements, lifters can maximize the benefits of resistance band training while minimizing the risk of injury. Proper form ensures that the targeted muscle groups are effectively engaged, and that the resistance provided by the bands is efficiently utilized.

Another fundamental concept we have emphasized is the principle of progressive overload. This involves gradually increasing the resistance level of the bands over time, allowing the body to adapt and grow stronger in response to the increased demand. By consistently challenging the muscles with higher levels of resistance, powerlifters can continue to make gains in strength and power, avoiding plateaus and ensuring ongoing progress.

Resistance bands can be particularly useful for providing assistance or added resistance during the three main powerlifting exercises: squats, deadlifts, and bench presses. By incorporating bands into these lifts, powerlifters can target specific muscle groups, improve joint stability, and enhance the overall quality of their movement patterns. For example, using bands during squats can help to emphasize glute and quadricep activation, while banded bench presses can increase tricep and chest engagement.

In addition to the main lifts, resistance bands can be utilized for a variety of accessory exercises

that complement powerlifting training. These exercises can help to address specific weaknesses, improve muscle imbalances, and promote overall structural balance. Some examples of effective accessory exercises

179

include banded glute bridges, pull-aparts, and face pulls.

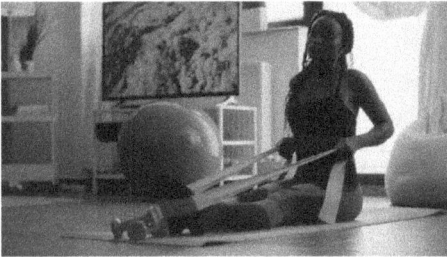

The benefits of incorporating resistance bands into a powerlifting routine are numerous and far-reaching. For beginners, resistance bands provide a safe and accessible way to build foundational strength and master proper form. As lifters progress, bands can be used to add variety to training, prevent stagnation, and target specific areas for improvement. Even experienced powerlifters can benefit from the unique challenges posed by resistance band training, using them to refine technique, overcome plateaus, and maintain joint health.

Beyond the physical benefits, training with resistance bands can also have positive mental and practical implications. The versatility and portability of bands make them an ideal option for lifters who travel frequently or have limited access to traditional gym equipment. They also provide a cost-effective alternative to expensive weightlifting machines and free weights. Mentally, the process of mastering new techniques and overcoming the challenges posed by resistance band training can foster a sense of accomplishment, boost confidence, and cultivate a growth mindset.

In summary, powerlifting with resistance bands is a highly effective and adaptable training approach that offers a wide range of benefits for lifters of all levels. By focusing on proper form, progressive overload, and targeted accessory work, powerlifters can harness the power of resistance bands to optimize their strength, power, and overall performance. The techniques and principles covered in this book provide a solid foundation for anyone looking to incorporate resistance band training into their powerlifting journey. With consistent practice, patience, and dedication, lifters can unlock their full potential and achieve their goals both in and out of the gym.

Setting Goals for Continued Progress in Powerlifting

Having a clear and well-defined set of goals is essential for any powerlifter looking to make consistent progress and achieve long-term success. When incorporating resistance bands into your training routine, setting specific, measurable, achievable, relevant, and time-bound (SMART) goals can help you stay focused, motivated, and accountable throughout your powerlifting journey.

The first step in setting effective goals is to conduct a thorough assessment of your current strengths and weaknesses. Take the time to honestly evaluate your lifting capabilities, technique, and overall performance. Identify areas where you excel and those that need improvement. This self-awareness will serve as the foundation for creating goals that are tailored to your unique needs and aspirations.

Once you have a clear understanding of your starting point, begin crafting specific goals for each aspect of your powerlifting training. These goals should be focused and well-defined, addressing particular lifts, muscle groups, or technical skills you wish to improve. For example, instead of setting a vague goal like "get stronger," aim for something more concrete such as "increase my banded deadlift one-rep max by 20 pounds in the next three months."

To ensure that your goals are measurable, establish clear benchmarks and tracking methods. This could involve keeping a detailed training log, recording videos of your lifts, or using a performance tracking app. By consistently monitoring your progress, you will be able to celebrate your victories, identify areas for improvement, and make data-driven adjustments to your training plan as needed.

When setting goals, it is crucial to strike a balance between ambition and realism. While it is important to challenge yourself and push beyond your comfort zone, setting goals that are too lofty or unrealistic can lead to frustration, burnout, and even injury. Consider factors such as your training experience, available time and resources, and individual rate of progress. Aim to set goals that are achievable with dedicated effort and consistent work, but that also require you to stretch and grow as a lifter.

Relevance is another key factor to consider when setting powerlifting goals. Your goals should align with your overall values, priorities, and long-term objectives. Ask yourself why each goal matters to you and how achieving it will contribute to your larger vision for your powerlifting journey. By setting goals that are personally meaningful and connected to your deeper motivations, you will be more likely to stay committed and persevere through challenges and setbacks.

Finally, make sure your goals are time-bound by assigning specific deadlines or target dates for achievement. Having a clear timeline creates a sense of urgency and helps you prioritize your efforts. Break larger goals down into smaller, more manageable milestones, and celebrate each incremental victory along the way. Regularly review and reassess your goals, adjusting as needed based on your progress, changing circumstances, or new insights gained through experience.

In addition to setting SMART goals, there are several other strategies you can employ to support your continued progress in powerlifting with resistance bands. First, seek out knowledge and guidance from experienced lifters, coaches, or training resources. Continuously educating yourself about proper form, programming, recovery, and nutrition will help you make

185

informed decisions and optimize your training approach.

Second, cultivate a dedicated support system of training partners, friends, and family members who understand and encourage your powerlifting pursuits. Surrounding yourself with positive influences and accountability partners can provide motivation, feedback, and camaraderie that will help you stay committed to your goals.

Third, embrace the power of consistency and discipline. Progress in powerlifting is rarely linear, and there will inevitably be difficulties along the way. By showing up consistently, putting in the work, and maintaining a growth mindset, you will be able to weather the challenges and continue making strides toward your goals.

Finally, remember to celebrate your victories, learn from your setbacks, and find joy in the process. Powerlifting is as much a mental game as it is a physical one, and maintaining a positive outlook and sense of perspective is essential for long-term success and fulfillment.

Setting goals for continued progress in powerlifting with resistance bands is a critical component of any lifter's journey. By crafting SMART goals, seeking knowledge and support, cultivating consistency and discipline, and maintaining a growth mindset, you will be well-equipped to navigate the challenges and triumphs of your powerlifting career. With clear intentions, strategic planning, and unwavering dedication, you can achieve remarkable progress and unlock your full potential as a powerlifter.

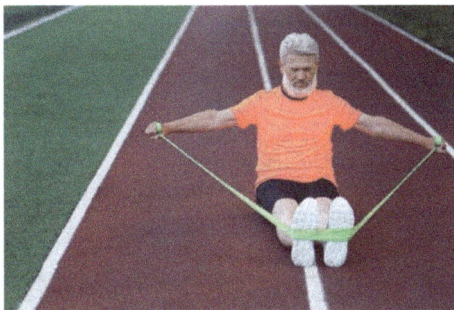

Resources for Further Learning and Training in Powerlifting with Resistance Bands

As you continue to explore and refine your powerlifting techniques with resistance bands, it is essential to have access to high-quality resources that can support your ongoing learning and skill development. Whether you are a beginner looking to build a solid foundation or an experienced lifter seeking to take your training to the next level, there is a wealth of information and guidance available to help you along your journey.

One of the most accessible and valuable resources for further learning is the vast array of online courses, tutorials, and educational content. Platforms like YouTube, Instagram, and dedicated fitness websites offer a treasure trove of videos and articles created by experienced powerlifters, coaches, and industry experts. These resources can provide in-depth demonstrations of proper form, detailed explanations of training principles, and step-by-step guides for incorporating resistance bands into your powerlifting routine.

When searching for online content, look for reputable sources with a proven record of accomplishment of providing accurate, evidence-based information. Seek out experienced practitioners who prioritize safety, technique, and long-term progress over flashy gimmicks or quick fixes. Be sure to cross-reference information from multiple sources and approach any new advice or techniques with a critical eye, always prioritizing your own health and well-being.

In addition to online resources, attending in-person workshops, seminars, and clinics can be an invaluable way to deepen your knowledge and refine your skills. Many gyms, powerlifting clubs, and fitness organizations offer specialized training events focused on resistance band techniques, programming, and performance optimization. These immersive learning experiences provide the opportunity to work directly with knowledgeable instructors, receive personalized feedback, and connect with like-minded lifters who share your passion for powerlifting.

When considering a workshop or seminar, research the credentials and reputation of the host organization and instructors. Look for events that offer a comprehensive curriculum, hands-on learning opportunities, and a supportive, inclusive environment. Do not be afraid to ask questions, seek clarification, and engage actively in the learning process. The insights and connections you gain from these experiences can be invaluable in shaping your ongoing powerlifting journey.

Books and print publications are another excellent resource for diving deeper into the world of powerlifting with resistance bands. There are numerous books available that cover topics ranging from basic technique and programming to advanced strategies for competitive performance. Look for titles written by respected coaches, athletes, and sports scientists who have a proven record of accomplishment of success in the field.

When selecting a book, consider your current skill level, specific training goals, and learning style. Some books may be more technical in nature, delving into the scientific principles behind resistance band training, while others may focus more on practical application and sample training programs. Read reviews, ask for recommendations from experienced lifters, and do not hesitate to preview a book's content before making a purchase to ensure it aligns with your needs and interests.

Another powerful resource for ongoing learning and support is the powerlifting community itself. Joining a local powerlifting club, participating in online forums, or engaging with social media groups dedicated to resistance band training can connect you with a wealth of knowledge, experience, and camaraderie. These communities provide a platform for sharing tips, asking questions, and learning from the successes and challenges of others who are on a similar journey.

When engaging with the powerlifting community, remember to approach interactions with an open mind, a respectful attitude, and a willingness to both learn and contribute. Be cautious of individuals who make exaggerated claims, promote dangerous practices, or engage in negativity or personal attacks. Surround yourself with supportive, knowledgeable, and ethical lifters who prioritize safety, sportsmanship, and the long-term health of the sport.

Finally, consider working with a qualified powerlifting coach or personal trainer who specializes in resistance band techniques. A skilled coach can provide personalized guidance, help you refine your form, and develop a customized training plan that aligns with your unique goals, abilities, and lifestyle. They can also offer accountability, motivation, and support as you navigate the difficulties of your powerlifting journey.

When selecting a coach, look for individuals with relevant certifications, a proven record of accomplishment of success, and a coaching philosophy that resonates with your values and goals. Schedule a consultation or trial session to ensure good fitness before committing to a long-term coaching relationship. Remember, a coach's role is to empower you with the knowledge, skills, and confidence to take ownership of your own training and progress.

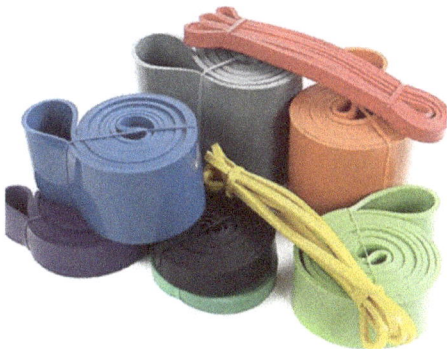

The path to mastering powerlifting with resistance bands is a continuous journey of learning, growth, and self-discovery. By leveraging the wealth of resources available – from online content and educational events to

books, communities, and coaching support – you can arm yourself with the knowledge and tools needed to achieve your full potential as a lifter. Embrace the process, stay curious, and never stop exploring the exciting possibilities that await you in the world of powerlifting with resistance bands.

Types of Bands

1. Pull-Up Bands (Loop Bands): Type we use for Power Lifting

   - Description: Large, continuous loop bands of various thicknesses and resistance levels.

- Uses:

  - Assisted pull-ups and chin-ups

  - Assisted dips

  - Powerlifting exercises (e.g., banded squats, deadlifts, bench press)

  - Stretching and mobility work

2. Tube Bands with Handles:

  - Description: Elastic tubes with handles attached to each end, available in different resistance levels.

  - Uses:

  - Upper body exercises (e.g., chest press, rows, shoulder press, bicep curls, tricep extensions)

- Lower body exercises (e.g., squats, lunges, leg abductions, leg extensions)

- Functional training and sports-specific movements

- Rehabilitation and physical therapy

3. Mini Loop Bands:

- Description: Small, circular bands that are typically 9-12 inches in diameter, available in various resistance levels.

- Uses:

- Lower body exercises (e.g., glute bridges, hip thrusts, lateral walks, clamshells)

- Upper body exercises (e.g., banded push-ups, pull-aparts, shoulder external rotations)

- Activation and warm-up exercises

- Physical therapy and rehabilitation

4. Therapy Bands (Flat Bands):

  - Description: Thin, flat sheets of elastic material, available in rolls or pre-cut lengths.

  - Uses:

    - Rehabilitation and physical therapy exercises

    - Stretching and mobility work

    - Low-intensity strength training

    - Posture correction and alignment exercises

5. Figure-8 Bands:

- Description: Elastic bands shaped like a figure-8, with loops on each end for foot and hand placement.

- Uses:

- Lower body exercises (e.g., leg extensions, leg curls, hip abductions)

- Upper body exercises (e.g., bicep curls, tricep extensions, lateral raises)

- Functional training and sports-specific movements

- Rehabilitation and physical therapy

6. Lateral Resistance Bands:

- Description: Short, flat bands with Velcro cuffs on each end, designed to provide lateral resistance.

- Uses:

  - Speed and agility training

  - Lateral movement exercises (e.g., lateral shuffles, lateral bounds)

  - Sports-specific training (e.g., skating, skiing, basketball defense)

  - Injury prevention and rehabilitation

7. Fabric Resistance Bands:

  - Description: Woven fabric bands that are typically gentler on the skin and more durable than latex bands.

  - Uses:

  - Upper body exercises (e.g., rows, chest press, shoulder press)

- Lower body exercises (e.g., squats, lunges, glute bridges)

- Stretching and mobility work

- Suitable for individuals with latex allergies

These are the main types of resistance bands; each designed to target specific muscle groups and support various training goals. When selecting resistance bands, consider your fitness level, the exercises you plan to perform, and any specific requirements, such as latex allergies or portability needs.

Remember to always inspect your bands for signs of wear and tear before use and replace them as needed to ensure your safety during workouts.

Let's face it – pull-ups are challenging for most people. According to a study conducted by the Human Performance Laboratory, "Many individuals struggle with being able to complete one repetition (rep) and increasing the maximum number of reps they can complete."

This is where the best pull-up assist bands come into play. With the right tools to support and challenge yourself appropriately, you can accurately monitor your progress towards your goals, whatever they may be. Pull-up assist bands allow users to develop the upper body muscles associated with completing unassisted pull-ups in an achievable manner.

GarageGym reviews tested over 100 resistance bands in the quest to find the best pull-up assistance bands available on the market. Let's dive right in.

7 Best Pull-Up Assist Bands

Best Pull-Up Assist Band Bundle: Fringe Sport Latex-Free Strength Bands

Best Pull-Up Assist Bands for Travel: INTENT SPORTS Pull-up Assist Bands – Assistance and Resistance Bands for Pull-Up

Best Pull-Up Assist Bands for Athletes: Gymreapers Resistance Pull-up Bands

Best Pull-Up Assist Bands for Beginners: SYNTECSO 220-440Lbs Pull-up Assistance Bands

Best Heavy-Duty Pull-Up Assist Bands: Rogue Monster Bands

Best Pull-Up Assist Single Band: Vulcan Resistance Band Light Strength Band

Best Pull-up Assistance Bands for Full Body Workout: Tikaton Pull-up Assist Bands Set

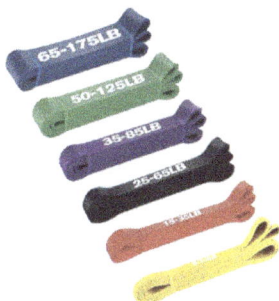

I Band Color I Resistance (lbs.) I Resistance (kg) I Suggested Use I

I Yellow   I 8-10   I 0.9-6.8   I
Beginners, rehabilitation, light assistance I

I Red   I 15-35   I 6.8-15.9   I
Beginners to intermediate, light to medium assistance I

I Black   I 25-65   I 27.2-56.7   I
Advanced, extra heavy assistance I

| Purple | 35-85 | 36.3-79.4 |
Advanced, ultra-heavy assistance |

| Green | 50-125 | 11.3-22.7 |
Intermediate, medium assistance |

| Blue | 65-175 | 18.1-36.3 |
Intermediate to advanced, heavy assistance |

| Orange | 100-200 | 45.4-90.7 |
Elite, maximum resistance | (not shown)

Please note that the resistance levels provided are estimates and can vary slightly depending on the brand and the length of the band. The suggested use is a general guideline, and the appropriate band color for you may vary based on your strength level and the specific exercise you are performing.

Resistance bands are typically rated for a specific weight or resistance level when stretched to a certain length, *often around 1.5 to 2 times their original length.* This is because the resistance of the band increases as it is stretched further.

When using resistance bands for pull-up training or any other exercise, it is essential to choose a band with an appropriate resistance level for your current strength and fitness goals. As you progress, you can gradually increase the resistance by using thicker bands or combining multiple bands to continue challenging your muscles.

When selecting a band for your pull-up or other exercises, consider the following factors:

1. Your current strength level and fitness goals

2. The number of unassisted repetitions you can perform

3. The specific exercise and the desired level of assistance or resistance

It is recommended to start with a band that provides enough assistance to allow you to perform the desired number of repetitions with proper form. As you progress and become stronger, you can gradually decrease the level of assistance by switching to a band with less resistance or combining multiple bands to fine-tune the resistance level.

Remember to always prioritize proper form and technique over the amount of resistance used. If you experience pain or discomfort during an exercise, stop and reassess your form or consider using a band with less resistance.

My personal Power Lifting Band workout:

Here is your modified Power Band Workout with more detail and the muscles each exercise targets:

Deadlift (Targets: Hamstrings, Glutes, Lower Back, Upper Back, Core)

Due to your hip concerns, you perform a lying deadlift with a blue band tied off between your feet. This variation allows you to maintain the same motion as a weighted deadlift while reducing the stress on your back and hips. By using the blue band, you can maintain a heavy resistance to effectively target your hamstrings, glutes, lower back, upper back, and core muscles.

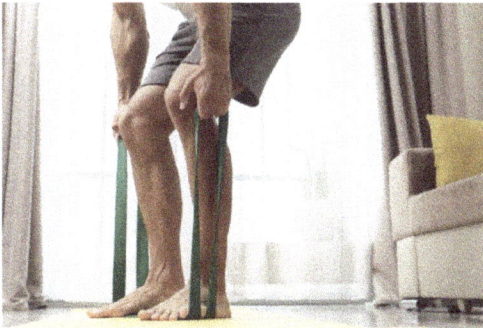

To perform the lying deadlift, lie on your back with your feet shoulder-width apart and the band secured between your feet. Grasp the band with both hands, keeping your arms straight. Engage your core and lift your hips off the ground, driving through your heels and squeezing your glutes at the top of the movement. Slowly lower your hips back to the starting position, maintaining tension in the band throughout the exercise.

Back Exercises

Overhead Pull-Downs (Targets: Latissimus Dorsi, Rear Deltoids, Biceps)

For overhead pull-downs, you alternate between the green and blue bands, depending on the desired intensity. This exercise primarily targets your latissimus dorsi (lats), the large muscles of your back that give you the "V-taper" look. It also engages your rear deltoids and biceps.

To perform overhead pull-downs, secure the band to a high anchor point. Grasp the band with both hands, palms facing away from you, and step back to create tension. Start with your arms extended overhead, then pull the band down towards your chest, squeezing your shoulder blades together. Slowly return to the starting position, maintaining control throughout the movement.

Low Rows (Targets: Middle Back, Rear Deltoids, Biceps)

Low rows target your middle back muscles, including the rhomboids and middle trapezius, as well as your rear deltoids and biceps. You use either the green or blue band for this exercise, allowing you to adjust the resistance based on your strength and goals.

To perform low rows, secure the band to a low anchor point. Grasp the band with both hands, palms facing each other, and step back to create tension. Start with your arms extended in front of you, then pull the band towards your abdomen, keeping your elbows close to your body. Squeeze your shoulder blades together at the end of the movement, then slowly return to the starting position.

Chest Exercises

Incline Bench Press (Targets: Upper Chest, Front Deltoids, Triceps)

The incline bench press primarily targets your upper chest muscles (the clavicular head of the pectoralis major), as well as your front deltoids and triceps. You use either the green or blue band for this exercise, allowing you to select the appropriate resistance level.

To perform the incline bench press, secure the band to a low anchor point and lie on an incline bench. Grasp the band with both hands, palms facing away from you, and position your hands slightly wider than shoulder-width apart. Press the band upwards, extending your arms fully, then slowly lower the band back to your chest.

Flat Bench Press (Targets: Middle and Lower Chest, Front Deltoids, Triceps)

The flat bench press targets your middle and lower chest muscles (the sternal head of the pectoralis major), as well as your front deltoids and triceps. As with the incline bench press, you use either the green or blue band, depending on your desired resistance level.

To perform the flat bench press, secure the band to a low anchor point and lie on a flat bench. Grasp the band with both hands, palms facing away from you, and position your hands slightly wider than shoulder-width apart. Press the band upwards, extending your arms fully, then slowly lower the band back to your chest.

Shoulder Exercises

Shoulder Press (Targets: Anterior Deltoids, Lateral Deltoids, Triceps)

The shoulder press is a compound exercise that primarily targets your anterior deltoids (the front part of your shoulder) and lateral deltoids (the side part of your shoulder). It also engages your triceps. You perform this exercise with a heavy resistance band to effectively challenge your shoulder muscles.

To perform the shoulder press, stand on the center of the band with your feet shoulder-width apart. Grasp the band with both hands, palms facing forward, and position your hands at shoulder level. Press the band overhead, extending your arms fully, then slowly lower the band back to shoulder level.

Side Lateral Raise (Targets: Lateral Deltoids, Supraspinatus)

The side lateral raise isolates your lateral deltoids, the muscles responsible for lifting your arms out to the side. It also targets the supraspinatus, one of the four rotator cuff muscles that stabilize your shoulder joint.

To perform the side lateral raise, stand on one end of the band with your feet shoulder-width apart. Grasp the other end of the band with your opposite hand, palm facing your thigh. Keep your arm straight and lift the band out to the side until your arm is parallel to the floor. Slowly lower the band back to the starting position. Repeat on the other side.

Triceps Exercises

Tricep Extensions (Targets: Triceps Brachii)

Tricep extensions effectively isolate and target all three heads of your triceps brachii (the

213

muscle on the back of your upper arm). You use the green band and focus on strict form, keeping your elbows tucked close to your body.

To perform tricep extensions, secure the band to a high anchor point. Grasp the band with both hands, palms facing each other, and step forward to create tension. Start with your elbows bent and your hands behind your head. Extend your arms fully, squeezing your triceps at the end of the movement, then slowly return to the starting position.

Tricep Pushdowns (Targets: Triceps Brachii)

Tricep pushdowns also target all three heads of your triceps brachii, helping to build strength and definition in the back of your arms. As with tricep extensions, you use the green band and focus on maintaining strict form throughout the exercise.

To perform tricep pushdowns, secure the band to a high anchor point. Grasp the band with both hands, palms facing down, and step forward to create tension. Start with your elbows bent at a

90-degree angle, keeping your upper arms close to your body. Push the band down, fully extending your arms, then slowly return to the starting position.

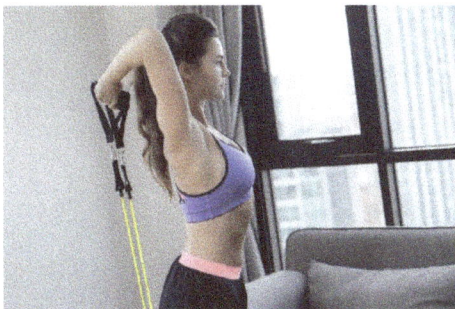

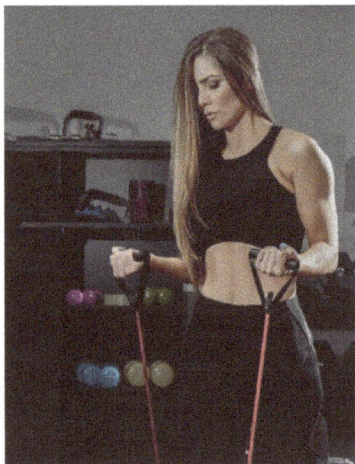

Bicep Exercises

Standing or Lying Bicep Curl (Targets: Biceps Brachii, Brachialis, Brachioradialis)

The standing or lying bicep curl targets the biceps brachii (the main muscle on the front of your upper arm), as well as the brachialis and brachioradialis (muscles that assist in elbow

216

flexion). You use the green band for this exercise, allowing you to focus on strict form and controlled movements.

To perform a standing bicep curl, stand on one end of the band with your feet shoulder-width apart. Grasp the other end of the band with your palm facing forward. Keep your upper arm stable and curl the band towards your shoulder, squeezing your bicep at the top of the movement. Slowly lower the band back to the starting position.

To perform a lying bicep curl, lie on your back with your feet shoulder-width apart and the band secured under your feet. Grasp the band with both hands, palms facing forward. Keep your upper arms stable and curl the band towards your shoulders, squeezing your biceps at the top of the movement. Slowly lower the band back to the starting position.

Hammer Curls (Targets: Biceps Brachii, Brachialis, Brachioradialis)

217

Hammer curls are a variation of the bicep curl that places more emphasis on the brachialis and brachioradialis muscles. You wrap the band around a bench and use either the green or blue band, depending on your desired resistance level.

To perform hammer curls, sit on a bench with the band wrapped around the base of the bench. Grasp the ends of the band with your palms facing each other. Keep your upper arms stable and curl the band towards your shoulders, maintaining a neutral wrist position throughout the movement. Slowly lower the band back to the starting position.

Squats (Targets: Quadriceps, Hamstrings, Glutes, Calves, Core)

Due to your back and hip surgeries, you limit your squats to twice a month and incorporate other leg exercises and cycling into your routine. When performing squats, you use the green band for a simple band squat and the purple band for wall squats.

To perform a simple band squat, stand on the center of the band with your feet shoulder-width apart. Grasp the ends of the band and position your hands at shoulder level. Lower your body into a squat position, keeping your chest up and your weight on your heels. Push through your heels to return to the starting position, squeezing your glutes at the top of the movement.

To perform a wall squat, secure the purple band to a low anchor point and position yourself against a wall with your feet shoulder-width apart. Place the band around your hips and step forward to create tension. Lower your body into a squat position, keeping your back pressed against the wall. Push through your heels to return to the starting position, squeezing your glutes at the top of the movement.

Face Pulls (Targets: Rear Deltoids, Middle Trapezius, Rhomboids, External Rotators)

Face pulls are one of your favorite exercises, as they help build strength in your rear deltoids and upper back muscles. You attach the purple band at eye level and perform 3 sets of face pulls at the beginning of your workout to loosen up your shoulders and chest.

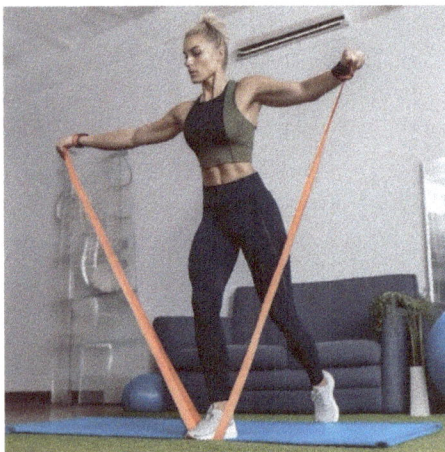

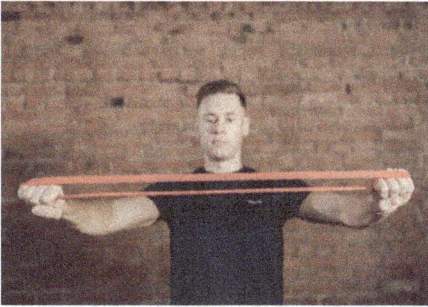

To perform face pulls, secure the band to a high anchor point at eye level. Grasp the ends of the band with both hands, palms facing each other. Step back to create tension, keeping your arms extended in front of you. Pull the band towards your face, keeping your elbows high and squeezing your shoulder blades together. Slowly return to the starting position, maintaining control throughout the movement.

In conclusion, your Power Band Workout effectively targets all major muscle groups using a combination of purple, green, and blue pull-up bands. By incorporating exercises like the lying deadlift, overhead pull-downs, low rows, bench presses, shoulder presses, lateral raises, tricep extensions, tricep pushdowns, bicep curls, hammer curls, squats, and face pulls, you can build strength, improve muscle definition, and enhance overall functional fitness.

Remember to focus on maintaining proper form, selecting the appropriate resistance level for each exercise, and listening to your body to avoid overexertion or injury. Consistently performing this well-rounded Power Band Workout, along with proper nutrition and recovery practices, can help you achieve your fitness goals and maintain a healthy, active lifestyle. Thanks for reading. Remember to look for my other Best-Selling Books HYSOMETRIC & HOLD THE POWER.

www.ingramcontent.com/pod-product-compliance
Lightning Source LLC
Chambersburg PA
CBHW051245020426
42333CB00025B/3054